Mind That Child

A Medical Memoir

Dr Simon Rowley
With Adam Dudding

16pt

Read How You Want
LARGE PRINT BOOKS, BRAILLE & DAISY

Copyright Page from the Original Book

PENGUIN

UK | USA | Canada | Ireland | Australia
India | New Zealand | South Africa | China

Penguin is an imprint of the Penguin Random House group of companies, whose addresses can be found at global.penguinrandomhouse.com.

Penguin
Random House
New Zealand

First published by Penguin Random House New Zealand, 2018

10 9 8 7 6 5 4 3 2 1

Cover and text design by Cat Taylor © Penguin Random House New Zealand
Cover illustration by Peter Hatter/Trevillion Images
Back cover photo © Simon Rowley
Prepress by Image Centre Group
Printed and bound in Australia by Griffin Press,
an Accredited ISO AS/NZS 14001 Environmental Management Systems Printer

A catalogue record for this book is available from the National Library of New Zealand.

ISBN 978-0-14-377198-2
eISBN 978-0-14-377199-9

penguin.co.nz

MIX
Paper from responsible sources
FSC
www.fsc.org
FSC™ C009448

NOTE ABOUT NAMES

To preserve the privacy of individuals I have changed most names as well as occasional identifying characteristics of the patients and parents whose stories appear in these pages. In a couple of places, details from real-life cases have been amalgamated to further blur identification.

TABLE OF CONTENTS

MIND THAT CHILD

Dr Simon Rowley is a senior consultant neonatologist at Auckland City Hospital (originally National Women's Hospital) with teaching links to Starship Children's Hospital. Training first in Dunedin and Christchurch, Rowley completed his postgraduate studies at the University of Oxford, UK. He also ran his own general paediatrics private practice in Auckland for 30 years, looking after children of all ages, and was visiting paediatrician for Plunket family centres over that same time. He is chair of the Paediatric Vocational Training Committee for the Auckland and Northern Region and a director of Physician Education.

Rowley is an honorary lecturer at the University of Auckland School of Medicine, and a recipient of the Dennis Pickup Clinical Educator Award (2014) and a Distinguished Clinical Teacher Award (2015).

One of Rowley's specialist areas is neonatal brain development, and he is both a trustee and presenter for the Brainwave Trust; others include early childhood behavioural and developmental outcomes, and medical ethics. In particular, he is interested in how we make decisions about end-of-life care in the vulnerable, sick or newborn infant.

He is married with four adult children and lives in Mt Eden, Auckland.

To my wife Ann, and our children –
Joe, Patrick, Tom and Francesca.

And to all the children and families
who have been part of this lifelong experience.

CHAPTER 1

WARD ROUND, THURSDAY EVENING

Today's ward round is an eventful one, but it's nothing out of the ordinary.

2

The baby is lying on her back. There are oxygen prongs up her nose and a drip connected to her bellybutton, but she seems calm and relaxed – not at all concerned as the ultrasonographer repeatedly passes the wand over her tummy while peering at the screen that's playing a grainy black and white movie of the child's insides. As the image is refocused and reframed, zoomed in and out, we can all see the intricate plumbing of the gut, and the heart chambers pumping like little fists clenching and unclenching.

The girl's father, a burly fellow in sweatpants and jandals, is watching from the other side of the table with the stunned expression I've seen before on parents on their first day in this ward – a combination of concern, confusion and exhaustion. To him, no doubt, his daughter looks tiny and vulnerable, but to the medical team she looks enormous because, unlike the majority of babies who end up in the level 3 Newborn Intensive Care Unit (NICU), she was born after a full-term pregnancy.

She needs NICU's specialised skills and multimillion-dollar equipment not because she's a preterm but because she has trisomy 21 – Down syndrome. As well as the mild to moderate intellectual disability and distinctive facial features caused by her extra chromosome, this means she faces a range of potential health problems, some life-threatening, and she may need swift surgery.

3

The picture emerging on the ultrasound monitor is partly good: a congenital heart defect often seen in babies with Down syndrome is not present. But there are signs of pulmonary hypertension, where high blood pressure in the lungs hinders the transfer of oxygen to the blood, turning the baby blue. Of even greater concern are blood results which suggest she is at risk of developing leukaemia in later childhood. The hospital haematologists are taking a close interest and making suggestions for future management.

Paediatric trainee Logan Wingate is the registrar responsible for the baby's care today, and as the ultrasound investigation continues he talks me through her statistics – blood pressure, oxygen saturation, heart rate, breathing patterns, electrolytes, blood sugars, body temperature, bowel motions, general appearance, milk-feed volumes – referring only occasionally to the columns of tiny figures in the baby's sheaf of notes.

His plan for the rest of the evening sounds about right to me: fluid restriction for hyponatraemia (low blood sodium); monitor the platelets for clotting; keep a close eye on blood pressure. But his suggestion to increase the volume of milk delivered to her stomach via a gastric tube sounds a bit ambitious – when your stomach's the size of a walnut, an extra few drops can cause discomfort and interfere with breathing. I suggest he instead aims for five millilitres. It's not exactly an order: whenever possible my role as consultant neonatal paediatrician isn't to boss the registrars around but rather guide them towards figuring things out themselves, but he nods and scribbles a quick note.

I ask the father if he's keeping on top of the growing mountain of information about his daughter's condition, and he smiles and nods but says he'd rather not have a full update until the mother returns. She's the one who'll want to hear all the technical details.

***

It's 4pm on a Thursday at Auckland City Hospital, and we're at the start of the evening ward round and handover. I will be the on-call consultant for the night, so I need to be brought up to date on the status of the 14 babies in the level 3 NICU.

These are the sickest babies – the ones who are extremely premature, or need assisted ventilation, or are fighting serious infections, or are recovering from abdominal surgery, or are awaiting heart surgery.

Over the course of 45 minutes Logan and two other NICU registrars, as well as a nurse specialist, lead me through the quiet, dimly lit wards. We try to match the lighting of the ward to the outside world, so the unit's lights are turned down even lower in the evening, with spotlights on the staff workstations. We keep our voices low too, though some fascinating recent research by Terri Inder, a Kiwi professor now in Boston, suggests that a bit of noise stimulation is good for the premature brain – and of course we also encourage parents to sing and talk to their babies.

There are only two babies per room, but they're swamped by a sprawling complex of equipment. Each lies in the centre of a $30,000 temperature-controlled incubator, tethered by a spaghetti of tubes and wires to monitors and an oxygen supply, and the bags of fluid, food and medicine that keep them alive. Their daily diet might include caffeine to regulate breathing, heparin to thin the blood, ibuprofen to repair a common circulatory malfunction, antibiotics to fight infection, morphine for post-operative pain, diuretics, glucose, proteins, probiotics, fat preparations and more.

At the head of each incubator there are knobs and dials and flashing lights, and a large computer screen that busily displays the accumulating data. Occasionally one of the machines emits a gentle chime to warn of a worrying oxygen saturation or heart rhythm or ventilator pressure. For the uninitiated it's rather like stumbling into the cockpit of a passenger jet during takeoff. For me, it's something like home.

***

Our little posse shuffles over to the ward's second baby. Again, Logan runs us through the numbers and outlines his plans. This baby has been fighting a serious infection as well as pulmonary hypertension. Scans conducted before birth suggested he might have problems with his brain, heart and gut, so we've had him in here for two weeks, getting him ready for surgery and investigating all his systems.

The good news is that his brain and heart are normal, and he should be OK for bowel surgery tomorrow. His numbers are good, but he also *looks* good.

For all our dependence on technology, there's still a lot of information you can collect about a child simply by watching for a few minutes. Medical data is encoded in the pinkness of skin, in the relative ease of breathing, in a facial expression. Preterm infants also manage to convey something of their personality even in those very early days. Their body – and especially their brain – is still under construction, but you can see the frame taking shape.

Some will motor around the incubator, putting their legs out of the portholes, and never remain still or in the same position. Others are quiet and don't explore their world much. Some resist nappy changes, much as a healthy full-term baby might. Others lie back, stretch and yawn and look bored with the world.

This child was born a month early so he's pretty small, but he's far from the smallest in the ward today. Later in the round we'll see a baby who was born days earlier at 23 weeks' gestation, weighing 550 grams. She's so small that if I placed her on my open hand with her feet on my wrist, you'd still see the tips of my fingers extending beyond her head.

Not that I'd dare do that: 23 weeks is on the absolute margin of survivability, and such a baby is extraordinarily fragile. Even changing a nappy can cause wide swings in cerebral blood pressure and trigger a brain haemorrhage, so we try to handle these tiny babies as gently and as infrequently as possible early on.

This particular 23-weeker is doing remarkably well all things considered, but I take care to tell the mother that it's best to think of this as a 'honeymoon period': all too often it is followed by worsening news as the extreme immaturity starts to declare itself and the complications begin.

It is difficult, but necessary, to keep parents' expectations realistic, because in a level 3 NICU baby things change fast. Half a century of rapid medical progress has turned a neonatal ward into a place of miracles, but it is still, and always will be, a place of death as well.

Take this evening.

As we're doing our ward round, the day-shift paediatric consultant who would normally join us is sitting with a family as intensive-care support for a newborn baby is withdrawn. Within a couple of hours the baby will be dead. This was another 23-weeker, born weighing less than 600 grams. Sometimes, when we know a baby is coming early, there's time to give the mother steroids and other drugs to fast-forward some foetal maturation processes, but this one came too fast. Since birth the baby has been struggling with immature lungs, heart enlargement and then infection, and was then found to have had a major cerebral haemorrhage with considerable brain destruction.

If the only thing that mattered here was lifespan we could stretch that out a little: we have machines to breathe for him, tubes to feed him, drugs to maintain some other bodily functions. But even if we pulled all the stops out, extreme disability is unavoidable, and death is all but certain, probably within days.

So now, after discussions between parents and medical staff, he has been taken off the path of ever more drastic interventions. He's been disconnected from the ventilator that was pushing moist air into failing lungs. The only medicine he's getting is a tiny dose of morphine to ensure there's no discomfort. Best of all, his family is with him, making the most of his final hours when they can see him for perhaps the first time without all those wires and needles and tubes and beeping monitors in the way.

As we pass the door, my colleague steps out to let us know about the family's decision and the baby's condition. The mood as we discuss the case is sombre, but businesslike.

There is a shared understanding that this decision is in the best interests of the child.

I ask my colleague if she has talked yet to the family about whether they will allow an autopsy. It's an opportunity to remind the young registrars that in around a third of cases, an autopsy adds new, valuable information about the causes of death. It can be very difficult to discuss an autopsy with parents and whānau when they are already in pain and distress, but we have to do it. Aside from the medical benefit, it's not uncommon, when parents return to see us later, for them to say they wish they'd had the courage to agree to the autopsy, so they could be clearer about why their baby died.

***

Moments like this are a reminder that there will always be a limit to what can be achieved in our wards.

In recent years the boundary between likely survival and likely death has been hovering around the 23- or 24-week mark. When I was a trainee intern in the early 1970s it was heartbreakingly higher. I remember vividly, at Rotorua Hospital, watching a beautiful baby boy born with immature lungs at 32 weeks' gestation struggle for breath for three days until he became exhausted and eventually died. The medical and nursing staff were able to give him fluids and oxygen, but otherwise we stood by helplessly. Just a few years later, we would know how to supply gas to his nose under pressure and save his life, and today a child of his gestational age and with the same degree of lung disease has virtually a 100 per cent chance of survival with minimal or no disability.

It has been gratifying, in my lifetime, to witness the transformation of this field of medicine, thanks to a series of research breakthroughs. The most notable was the discovery in the 1970s by New Zealand researchers that if you gave corticosteroids to a mother 12 hours before birth, you could accelerate foetal lung maturation. Later came breakthroughs in ventilation, the invention of artificial lung surfactant, blood transfusions, and refinements to reduce side effects that plagued early cohorts of premature survivors, such as eye damage from too much oxygen (this is what caused Stevie Wonder's blindness) and lung damage from tube ventilation.

Around the world, a handful of babies born before 23 weeks have survived without serious disability, and as-yet undreamed-of technologies may nudge the number even higher. But the paradox of modern neonatology is that each time a new method is found for keeping younger babies alive, a practitioner like me has to think more deeply about the benefits of chosing *not* to do so.

If you work in an NICU ward, this isn't some abstract philosophical question. As we keep pushing the limits, we mustn't forget that there is also a limit to what you can put a baby through.

***

By the time we finish the round, we've seen a baby who's had a stretch of gangrenous intestine surgically removed and may need to lose more, which risks leaving her with insufficient gut to survive without the misery of a lifetime of intravenous nutrition.

We've seen two babies with major congenital heart defects who have been referred to Auckland from out of town and are being readied for surgery.

Later, a baby who had seemed perfectly stable suddenly develops a distended tummy and becomes extremely sick. The mother is devastated and we have an awkward conversation: she had thought everything was going well, but by the end of the conversation she's in tears. The baby is likely to survive, but it will be a long road to recovery after this setback.

Today's ward round is an eventful one, but it's nothing out of the ordinary. Reading back through my account I can't help noticing how many times I've had to use the words 'died' or 'death'. I imagine that from the outside this evening's work could appear depressing or overwhelming – but curiously, that's not the case at all.

Working in the shadow of death and disability is certainly a heavy responsibility, and at times things can seem dark. Parts of this job are sad, of course, and it would be a rare neonatologist who hasn't cried at work more than once (and if they haven't, that's probably a problem).

But the joys of this work are also huge. It's hard to beat the feeling when parents bring a baby in months after discharge, and instead of a vulnerable little creature you're looking at a healthy baby and happy parents. I'm delighted every time someone stops me in the street and says 'You looked after my baby' – though when I ask 'How old is the baby now?' it's alarming how frequently the answer is 'Oh, he just turned 18' – or 25, or even older.

Five years ago I was honoured to be invited to the 21st birthday party of a young man whom I first met when he was a 23-week pretermer – the youngest baby we'd ever managed to save at that time. Later I heard that he had saved a young boy from drowning in a local swimming hole that summer. For me there was a satisfying symmetry in that story of life versus death.

By the end of this round I feel I have enough information to help me make decisions during the night; and, rather than feeling despondent, this fundamental routine of hospital life has left me feeling energised. It strikes me that half a century after I first decided I might like to study medicine, I'm still getting a kick out of it.

I'm 69 and in pretty good health, especially since I got a couple of replacement hips installed (and I think it did me some good to experience the medical system from the other end of the stethoscope). My duties at Auckland City Hospital, where I'm one of a team of eight specialists working alongside 16 registrars and nurse specialists, takes only 40 hours a week, which feels something like semi-retirement considering that until 18 months ago I was doing an additional 15 hours a week in my private paediatric practice.

I'm in no hurry to give up the neonatal work, though. There is always a challenging case or something I have never seen before. There is always a baby for whom you can feel happy at what they have achieved, or sad when things go wrong. There are always parents to help through an incredible journey, and a junior staff member who is keen to learn and to whom you can pass on some of your wisdom. I am, I know, a very lucky man.

CHAPTER 2

ALL THUMBS

It was at about this point in my career that I decided I definitely didn't want to be a surgeon.

The thumb didn't look right.

I'd done my best for the labourer whose left hand had been mangled in an accident on a north London construction site. I'd cut away the edges of injured tissue and cleaned the wound to reduce the chance of infection. But the next step – doing the delicate sutures required to repair the severed tendons of the thumb – was beyond my limited skills. I phoned the orthopaedic registrar and asked him to come down to the emergency department of this small district hospital in Harrow on the Hill to complete the tendon repair.

It's not for nothing that some surgeons have a reputation for arrogance, and this one clearly didn't feel like taking direction from a house surgeon not long out of some medical school in the distant Antipodes. He told me to sort it out myself. I glanced at the labourer – I still remember that his last name was Patel. He was in some discomfort but he hadn't noticed my anxiety, and his expression was trusting. I exchanged a look with the nurse assisting me and picked up my suture thread and needle.

It was at about this point in my career that I decided I definitely didn't want to be a surgeon.

***

My decision to be a doctor, of whatever brand, started with a sneeze.

I grew up on a sheep farm in south Otago, where my older brother Philip and I had a couple of cows to milk and were expected to shift sheep, bale or rake hay and help with the shearing, crutching and dipping. We'd practise driving the truck as we took out the smoko to the adult workers or when running errands to town.

One summer, when I was about 12, raking the hay left me with streaming eyes and constant sneezing, so I was taken to the local GP to see if he could help. After hearing my symptoms, he asked if my eyes were also itchy, and I was astounded that he could have known this without being told. How clever! It was my first introduction to the art of diagnosis, and I was intrigued.

I was equally impressed when, during a school holiday visit to cousins in Wanaka, I developed a stabbing chest pain that got worse with each intake of breath. I decided I was dying, but the local GP, Dr Blanc, a portly and kind man who reminded me of Hercules Poirot, noted my fever and told my aunt I had 'devil's grip' – a coxsackievirus infection for which his remedy was aspirin and bed rest.

From the age of 11, I was a boarder at John McGlashan College in Dunedin. At first I was bullied and terribly lonely, but eventually I settled in and thrived. There I met another impressive GP, Dr Borrie, who could drain an ear abscess or a swollen scrotum, burn off warts and excise verrucas, and repair most schoolboy injuries. When he heard I was thinking about studying medicine he took me along to watch him do a tonsillectomy.

My ambition was further fostered by the BBC TV series *Dr Finlay's Casebook*, which gave the impression that there were few jobs finer than being a charming country GP who provides a cradle-to-grave service to the inhabitants of a remote Scottish community. But it wasn't until my final year of school that the idea of medicine really began to gel, and it had a lot to do with my mother Joyce.

My mother had always wanted to go to university, but World War Two put an end to that and she joined the WAAF. She met my father, married in uniform and became a farmer's wife. All she really wanted to do was live in a big city like New York, in a whirl of high fashion, nights at the ballet and opera, and sipping cocktails overlooking the park. Instead she found herself behind a tractor on a drill sowing swedes, or making scones and afternoon cuppas for the farmhands. My decision to go to university was a fulfilment for her as much as for me.

I got off to a very shaky start. In my last year at school, having set my sights on medicine, I had to drop the language subjects I loved and take up physics and chemistry, neither of which interested me all that much.

My first year at Otago University was medical intermediate, but instead of focusing on the science papers I found either difficult or dull, I took advantage of my newfound freedom after the constraints of boarding school; there was a lot of partying and drinking and not a lot of study. The outcome is burned into my memory in quite a literal way: to this day, whenever I smell the scent of flowering azaleas it recalls exam time in Dunedin in 1966, and the dread I felt walking through the Botanic Gardens towards an exam I knew I wasn't prepared for.

In the end I scraped through all the papers, but my marks weren't good enough for medical school and I had to repeat the intermediate year. This time I worked extremely hard and got the grades I needed. Five years later, in 1972, I graduated MBChB. There is a photograph of me with my grandmother that day, with my wavy shoulder-length hair making me look like a King Charles spaniel.

In medicine, you gain hospital experience before you graduate, and conversely you continue to learn new skills long after you've formally joined the workforce. Which means that there can be a scarily long overlap where you have big responsibilities but don't necessarily know what you're doing.

At the end of my fifth year, with a year of undergraduate study still to come, I was asked by the superintendent of Balclutha Hospital if I'd like to cover the 'house officer' duties for a couple of weeks over the holidays.

Balclutha is the major service town for South Otago, and this was the very hospital where I was born 24 years earlier (after a labour induced at 36 weeks because the GP/obstetrician wanted to go on holiday, an outrageous and risky act of medical arrogance that no one would get away with these days). I was a local. I jumped at the chance.

I hadn't fully realised the seriousness of the role: I was dropped into the thick of clinical medicine, covering all the wards night and day. It was both exciting and terrifying. Exciting because I knew that I would learn how to suture, how to set fractures and how to insert intravenous infusions and prescribe medication. Terrifying because I quickly realised there wasn't going to be time to practise newly taught skills under supervision and become proficient before I was let loose on the unsuspecting public. I struggled, but was helped by the nursing staff who saw my inexperience and were kind enough not to roll their eyes whenever *they* saved the day and *I* got the credit.

Early one morning, in an incident that foreshadowed my adventure with Mr Patel's thumb, I was called to attend to a young woman who'd been in a car crash and had a massive facial laceration that needed suturing. I rang the boss, but he told me just to get on with it.

After a very long time – maybe an hour and a half – I had managed to suture the wound, leaving a huge scar with 30-odd stitches across the young woman's forehead. The next morning my senior's only comment was that I could have used more sutures. For years afterwards I worried that this woman would have a disfiguring scar that a plastic surgeon would have made light work of.

I admitted people with heart attacks in the middle of the night, treated acute asthmatic attacks, set fractures of the wrist, did my own wet-plate X-rays and, even worse, interpreted them, and helped women deliver mid-trimester miscarriages – infants born after the 24th week, which nowadays we would regard as viable.

Soon after this, as a trainee intern in Rotorua hospital, I did my first lumbar puncture (spinal tap) – on a three-month-old child. This involves carefully inserting a needle between two vertebrae in the lower back to puncture the fluid-filled space surrounding the spinal cord and withdraw a sample. Under normal circumstances the fluid is perfectly clear, but in this case it was thick yellow pus. This was obviously meningitis (a kind that's now rare, thanks to immunisation) – and devastating in its effects. The child survived but developed palsy of the eye muscles and went deaf.

The sight of purulent material oozing from a child's back left me woozy, but my reaction to the sight of blood was even worse. During one especially bloody procedure at Rotorua – suturing up a thigh wound – I fainted. It was Christmas Day, I was tired and most likely hungover, and the task involved sitting on a stool for an hour or so in a hot gown, stitching into a huge open wound with exposed inner veins and gristle. As I blacked out I dropped my utensils and slipped off the stool, but the wonderful nurses nearby saved me from hitting the floor, then brought me some water and cheered me up so that I was able to finish the grisly job.

***

My first placement after graduation, as a real, qualified doctor, was at Wellington Hospital in 1973 as a house surgeon. As a newbie I was rotated around the departments, starting with ophthalmology, which I loved – the exquisite intricacies of the eye; the beautiful equipment that was used for looking at them; the quick rewards if you were inspecting a patient who was in agony and spotted the foreign body, a wood chip, say, and were able to whip it out to provide instant, magical relief.

One of the more sobering jobs of the house surgeon was to ask the family of a newly deceased person if we could take the corneas from the eyes for transplants. It was tough on the grieving family, and not exactly easy for an inexperienced new doctor in his mid twenties. These days we would expect a senior member of staff to handle those difficult conversations with families, and junior staff would learn by quietly observing those interactions.

Even worse was trekking off to the mortuary on my own to retrieve an eye. More often than not it would be in the middle of the night, and I'd usually be on my own. Standing dissecting a dead person in a cold room surrounded by white-draped corpses on silver table slabs felt distinctly gothic.

In that first year at Wellington Hospital I worked rosters with up to 19 days' work in a row. I was constantly tired. But every new rotation as a house surgeon was exciting or interesting in its own way.

Adult medicine was often frantic. One night, another house surgeon and I had just given up resuscitating a man admitted with a heart attack when we were called to another crisis, and then another. Three hours later a volunteer helping the man's wife asked how we were getting on and I slumped into a chair in hysterical laughter and near-tears, wondering how I could break the news that he'd actually died three hours earlier, and we'd been so busy we'd forgotten to tell his relatives.

It was when I was assigned a three-month stint in the paediatric wards that I finally felt I had found my calling.

Hospital paediatrics covers an unusually broad range of medical situations, from broken bones to eye injuries, from infectious diseases to cancers, and naturally the department had to work closely with specialists from other areas. But there are many clinical areas that are unique to paediatrics – from treatment of premature babies and diagnosis of genetic disorders, to dealing with the unusual accidents children seem to specialise in such as coin-swallowing, poking things up their noses and falling out of trees.

For me what was especially rewarding was the interactions with kids. I enjoyed their quirky behaviours, their vulnerabilities and their honesty. I marvelled at the way they expressed their fear, joy and happiness all in the same moment. It was emotionally rewarding to try to help them through their hospital stay, and part of this was engaging not only with them but with their parents. I learnt how to pick up on parental anxiety, and could see it being transmitted directly to the child. Conversely, if the parents could be calm and reassuring, then half the battle was over.

The challenge of diagnosis and treatment was intellectually satisfying, but I also hugely enjoyed playing with the children, and in a clinical setting that's not an indulgence or a waste of time – it's an effective way of minimising trauma for the child. Some vital medical skills aren't really taught at medical school, and patience is one of them. Instead, you pick it up on the job by observing, or being mentored by, the best of your senior colleagues.

I realised that with paediatrics, you're never dealing with just one patient – the child – but with an entire whānau. You need to understand the parents' circumstances and the health of other family members, and sometimes you need to read between the lines to figure out things the child is unable to articulate.

I would find that there would be more to a sick or injured child than meets the eye. A child who has accidentally swallowed poison may turn out to be a child with ADHD whose parents have become too exhausted to monitor his every move, and they really need help with that.

I learnt that spending 10 or 20 minutes with the parents, getting their child's history and then chatting about anything from the latest rugby results to what school their child would go to, is all productive. In that time, while nothing much seems to be happening, the child relaxes and picks up that you are not the enemy. They are then much more likely to talk to you and even let you examine them without fuss.

Official training teaches us to examine a child on a flat surface, and to approach them from their right side; but I learnt that you'll get far more information from a young child if they are allowed to lie back on their parent's knees while you quietly palpate and listen and look at their abdomen, chest, mouth and ears.

Medical training takes a lifetime, and it would be another decade before I completed the last of my formal paediatric qualifications to become a Fellow of the Royal Australasian College of

Physicians. During that time I held a succession of positions in hospitals in New Zealand and the United Kingdom, squeezed in some travel, fell in love and got married. But it was during that first year in Wellington that the die was cast: I was going to be a doctor who worked with children.

***

By my mid thirties I found myself in Oxford, lecturing and practising child and adolescent psychiatry. I thought that perhaps this would be the area I would focus on for the rest of my career.

I enjoyed the adolescent work immensely. I played tennis with anorexic girls who would turn up with huge cakes that they had baked for me but would never eat themselves. I spent time talking to kids who were refusing to go to school, and realised that sometimes they were responding to subliminal messages from their parents, who felt better when the kid stayed home.

I did occasional school visits, including to the exclusive boarding and day-school Marlborough College in Wiltshire, the alma mater of government ministers, bank chairmen, archbishops, generals and minor royals, not to mention the communist spy Anthony Blunt and the singer Chris de Burgh.

One day I was asked to meet and assess a 17-year-old boy who dressed in a black cape and spent hours visiting churchyards and burial places, where he would read the poetry of Shelley and Keats. Perhaps, the teaching staff worried, all these morbid obsessions meant he was suicidal.

Over several interviews I established that he had no intention of harming himself; rather, he was indulging in an adolescent fantasy triggered initially by a six-month period of enforced bed rest because of an orthopaedic problem. I couldn't help thinking, though, that his curious behaviour could have been connected to the school environment itself: the grounds were like parks and the buildings were extravagantly grand, with interiors of elaborately carved wood and stained-glass windows designed by William Morris (another old Melburnian). Surrounded by such gothic splendour, no wonder the boy found it easy to slip into a fantasy world. A couple of years ago I spotted his name on LinkedIn and wrote to him; he's now director of a large UK company with sons of his own. He recalled our meetings and reflected – quite accurately I thought – on his adolescent hiccup.

After a year in this job, though, I realised I was missing working with younger children and babies, and I refocused my attention away from psychiatry and back to acute clinical paediatrics.

Whether working as a psychiatrist or as a neonatal doctor, I discovered something that bothered me a lot. My efforts to bring relief as a doctor would on occasion be totally overwhelmed by forces outside my control – the effects of poverty and social deprivation. When you're a psychiatrist looking for the causes of a child's major behavioural problems, sometimes the answer is painfully obvious: the extreme stress in the lives of the child's parents – or, as is commonly the case, single parent. When someone is struggling to cope with day-to-day life and isn't getting the social or financial support they need, it's hardly surprising that their child might start acting out or missing school or appearing unhappy.

In neonatal paediatrics, too, the impact of socioeconomics is stark. Poverty is a strong contributory factor towards a mother having a premature baby in the first place, and the poorer the mother, the less likely she is to have received adequate antenatal care.

The job of a neonatal unit is to maximise a baby's developmental outcomes, but once babies leave our care, what matters most is the quality of the environment they're discharged into. This effect is so large that researchers studying the impact of various neonatal interventions – different drugs, different types of ventilation, different feeding strategies and so on – have learnt that if you don't account for socioeconomic status in your analysis, it's impossible to make sense of the statistics.

I sometimes can't help thinking as we discharge a baby after four months' care, having spent the best part of a quarter of a million dollars on them, that perhaps we could be spending a bit more on improving the lives of the parents who will be looking after this child for the next 20 years.

Indeed, this is one of the motivations behind writing this book. My decades in the job have given me the perspective, and perhaps the right, to make a few observations about the choices we make if we want to improve the lives of the least fortunate among us.

You only need to read the newspaper to know that even in a rich country like New Zealand there are direct health consequences of financial and social disadvantage: children whose asthma is a direct result of growing up in a cold and mouldy home; shocking rates of rheumatic fever among Māori and Pasifika people due to crowded housing and poor access to primary healthcare. And it's not only children who are affected: being poor puts you at greater risk of obesity, diabetes, poor oral health, heart disease and stroke.

From early on I found it frustrating to see the limits of what can be achieved by medical means alone, and I knew I would never be a politician or activist. Over the years I've done what I can, but it was only relatively late in the piece that I became part of a science communication project that is, I believe, bringing about serious change in the way New Zealand thinks about social deprivation: in the early 2000s I became a trustee of the Brainwave Trust, a charity that focuses on the burgeoning field of child brain development.

In recent years we've gained a far more detailed understanding of the lifelong impact of bad childhood experiences – and the devastating effects these can have on brain development and physical health. A tough childhood – whether that's abuse, exposure to drugs and alcohol, or having a parent who's in jail or suffers from a psychiatric disorder – literally makes you less likely to end up a healthy adult.

Brainwave takes that science and spreads the word. We work with parents and policymakers, with youth court judges and prison inmates, with schoolchildren and teachers.

Some of the research findings we're sharing might seem blindingly obvious – it's been proven, for example, that a child who is consistently hugged and treated with tenderness will grow up to be happier, smarter, healthier and more successful than one who misses out. Yet these insights, and the interventions that they point to, have the potential to help New Zealand society make some of the steps needed to reduce childhood abuse and neglect, and create intergenerational change.

***

A few years after my decision to pull back from psychiatry and refocus on acute neonatal care, I was appointed as a consultant neonatal paediatrician at National Women's Hospital in Greenlane, Auckland. That's the same role I hold 31 years later, even though the hospital's name, location and structure have changed around me – NICU is now located in the Auckland City Hospital building in Grafton and comes under the aegis of Starship Children's Hospital, whose main building is next door.

That's why a lot of this book relates to my work caring for the smallest and sickest babies in a public hospital, and the teaching work that goes along with that – the view from the neonatal ward, if you like.

For almost accidental reasons I have had a secondary career for those 31 years. When I first took the hospital consultant role, the post wasn't quite full-time; this meant I was able to set up my own private paediatric practice in parallel, from an office in Remuera, working with children of all ages up to their late teens. The private work filled out my working week and topped up my income, but it also meant I stayed intimately connected to the broader journey of childhood development, rather than merely farewelling babies from neonatal intensive care.

It also meant that I've been in the box seat as the world of medicine – and society at large – has grappled with the recent apparent epidemics of child behavioural issues such as attention deficit and hyperactivity disorder (ADHD) and autism spectrum disorders (ASD). Later I'll talk about what I've learnt during an era of dizzying change and pharmacological 'miracle' cures, and some of the advice I've offered struggling parents over the years. I'll also look at issues such as foetal alcohol syndrome, developmental delay and cerebral palsy.

One of the reasons I love medicine as much as I do is that you never stop learning. Some of that's formal: if you don't keep up with the latest research, read the peer-reviewed journals and attend the international conferences, you're letting your patients down (and in the age of Google, they're much more likely to spot any gaps in your knowledge).

Some of the greatest lessons come when you least expect or want them – and I'll address some of those. I'll talk about the near-fatal accident involving one of my own children, and how it changed the way I approached being a paediatrician. And I'll talk about the time when my colleagues and I came to the horrifying realisation that a treatment designed to help the premature babies in our wards was in fact severely damaging some of them.

***

A doctor is always asking questions: What is wrong with this patient? How do I know I've made the right diagnosis? How can I best solve this problem? Is there a better way?

Sometimes, fortunately, the answer to that last question is yes.

Back in that London casualty department with Mr Patel and his injured thumb, I realised that even though I would never be a great surgeon, and even though the colleague who should have been coming to help me with the tendons would never arrive, there was another solution that might work for everybody.

Rather than ruin the thumb forever with a botched tendon repair, I took my needle and sewed up the skin and other tissues, leaving the tendons for a follow-up operation by someone more skilful in six weeks, by which time the inflamed tissues would have settled down. This was an accepted alternative approach for dirty wounds like this one, and had the advantage of slightly reducing the risk of infection.

My temporary patch-up went pretty well; but when I inspected my handiwork, it looked like I'd sewn it back on the wrong way round – the lack of attached tendons meant the thumb was flopping around loosely on poor Mr Patel's palm. The staff nurse and I exchanged another look, then we quickly bandaged up the hand into a semblance of the correct anatomical appearance and sent him on his way.

CHAPTER 3

A DETECTIVE IN THE NEONATAL UNIT

In an NICU, every moment of a neonate's life is meticulously recorded, from a nappy change to a major operation.

In 1994 my colleagues and I started to notice something very disturbing in our unit. Over one to two years we had seen close to a dozen babies in NICU with a very unusual brain injury that was causing disability and, in some cases, death.

These were all tiny babies, many of them under 1000 grams at birth, so, as harsh as it may sound, some incidence of disability and death was accepted – even though the medical skills at National Women's NICU and at others around the world had been improving in leaps and bounds. (In 1974 nine out of 10 babies born under 1000 grams at National Women's died; by 1994, eight out of 10 were surviving.)

Brain bleeds are not uncommon among the smallest of premature babies. This is why we routinely perform cranial ultrasounds, where you place the probe over the baby's fontanelle – the soft bit at the top of the head where the bones haven't as yet joined up – and take a peek inside the brain, looking for the telltale brighter areas where the soundwaves bounce more readily off a blood clot.

But as well as the 'ventricular' bleeds common to preterm infants, we were finding a small number of major 'intracerebral' haemorrhages, a type more commonly seen in adults with strokes. The bleeds were nearer the edges of the brain than the usual bleeds, and had a distinctive wedge shape on the brain scans.

Clearly something was going on, but we had no idea what.

One day after 'journal club' (that's where a group of doctors get together to discuss a recent article from a medical journal), a few of us discussed what might be happening, and our colleague Jane Harding, now a distinguished professor at the University of Auckland, offered to turn detective – not so much gumshoe with a magnifying glass as medico-scientific sleuth with a good head for numbers.

In an NICU, every moment of a neonate's life is meticulously recorded, from a nappy change to a major operation. This meant Harding could perform an elegant retrospective investigation known as a case control study. For every baby who had a mystery brain bleed, Harding identified babies born around the same time at a similar weight and gestational age who *hadn't* got sick. Using statistical techniques to compare 11 babies with severe brain injury against 22 controls without injury, she would theoretically be able to identify the risk factors associated with the injuries.

Theoretically – but the study didn't seem to work.

Harding plugged in the numbers for 50 different factors that might conceivably be relevant: the type of ventilation used on the baby; whether there had been infection or low blood pressure; whether the baby had also had one of the more common ventricular brain bleeds. But the data revealed little of significance. There was a weak association between the injuries and low blood pressure, but even that didn't make much sense, seeing as low blood pressure had been around since the dawn of time while the mystery bleeds had appeared only in the past two years.

Mystery unsolved, Harding wrote up her findings anyway, and presented them at a local meeting of neonatal and general paediatricians, asking everyone present if they had any thoughts on possible causes. The answer was a unanimous no.

But then – a stroke of luck. A few days later, a general paediatrician who'd been at the meeting came back to Harding to say he'd been thumbing through a medical journal and had seen an article about a neonatal unit in Birmingham which, in 1992, had seen a flurry of exactly the same rare brain bleeds. The article didn't, however, say what happened next, or if the Brits had found the cause.

Harding picked up the phone to the United Kingdom and talked to the article's author. She was told the Birmingham hospital had decided the injuries were probably connected to a common treatment known as 'chest physiotherapy'. They hadn't done a formal study or published their suspicions: they'd simply stopped the treatment and the bleeds stopped.

I was on call at NICU when Harding and the then head of department, David Knight, phoned me with this shocking piece of information. My first response was a loud 'Oh my god.' I was shocked, then on reflection felt ambivalent about the news: if it turned out to be true, and chest physiotherapy was the culprit, that meant we were responsible for these injuries. Yet it also meant there was something we could do about it right away. After I had put the phone down, one of us walked to the nursery and quietly announced an immediate halt to chest physiotherapy on the babies.

Harding quickly reran the calculations for her case control study, this time entering chest physiotherapy as a variable. To everyone's horror this confirmed the suspicion: those babies in our unit who had suffered the brain injuries had received far more – around four times as many – physiotherapy treatments than those who hadn't suffered an injury.

We immediately contacted all the other neonatal units in Australia and New Zealand, most of which were also using chest physiotherapy. At the same time we made arrangements to visit all the families of the affected babies: a total of 13 had been affected by the brain bleeds, and of those five had died.

We suddenly found ourselves in the middle of a controversial and very public incident, complete with a formal inquiry, disciplinary investigations and a degree of media hype. One academic would later refer to Harding's study as 'a fine piece of detective work', but perhaps unsurprisingly that's not how the babies' parents saw it. One father later described the inquiry as 'a whitewash'.

I will get to all that, but in order to fully understand how it's even possible that an NICU could end up harming children instead of healing them, I think it's helpful to first take a short tour through a history of neonatal medicine.

***

Modern neonatal care as we recognise it now really only began in the 1950s, but the first tentative steps towards systematic treatment of sick babies were made 70 years earlier. In the 1880s obstetrician Stéphane Tarnier began trialling infant incubators at a maternity hospital in Paris. The design was inspired by a poultry incubator – essentially a wooden box with a glass lid. Tarnier found that keeping the babies in a warm, humid and clean environment reduced infant mortality at the hospital by almost a third over three years. It reminded me of how, in winter on our farm in Otago, my father, my brother and I would bring motherless lambs into the kitchen and put them in a warm oven for several hours in a cardboard box with a dry blanket. These near-dead lambs would make a miraculous recovery. Incubators are the ideal 'oven' when dealing with tiny babies.

If a baby of any gestation is born unexpectedly at home, in a taxi or, say, in a GP's office, they invariably come in with hypothermia.

All that is needed is to dry the baby, discard the inevitable wet blanket and put the baby skin-to-skin on the mother's chest, covered with a warm, dry blanket – yet this is seldom done completely: the most common omission is a failure to discard the wet blanket, which increases heat loss. When babies get cold their metabolic requirements increase exponentially with each degree of fall in temperature, and then their blood sugar level falls.

Word spread of the amazing benefits of keeping small babies in a warmed box. At the Great Industrial Exposition of Berlin in 1896, Tarnier's colleague Martin Couney brought along six incubators and borrowed six premature babies from a Berlin hospital to put in them. Ordinarily none of the babies would have been expected to live, but all six survived. Over the next few years Couney's incubator babies became a kind of public entertainment: he displayed incubators at the 1897 Victorian Era Exhibition in Earl's Court, London and at similar expos in Nebraska and Paris, then at the 1901 Pan-American Exposition in Buffalo, New York. Eventually he set up a permanent incubator display at Luna Park on Coney Island, New York. It's hard to believe now, but parents would bring in their sickly babies to be treated for free, and visitors would pay 25 cents to take a look. The display ran until 1943 when Couney retired; he had earlier said he wouldn't stop until public hospitals set up their own dedicated incubator wards.

There was a slow but steady acceptance in the early 20th century of the idea that premature and sickly babies could and should be kept alive. Doctors and nurses began to specialise in neonatal care. Incubators grew more sophisticated and were increasingly pumped with oxygen, on the assumption that this would make breathing easier for babies with immature lungs.

Unfortunately, the use of pure oxygen became an early, devastating example of how a lifesaving idea can be flawed: oxygen certainly helped reduce rates of death and cerebral palsy but, from the 1940s on, doctors noticed many premature babies were developing a condition called retinopathy of prematurity, where abnormal blood vessels grew in the retina causing retinal detachment and blindness. It took researchers a long time to figure out that oxygen therapy was to blame, and longer still to figure out dosages of oxygen that would keep babies alive but not blind them. As recently as 1998, new research cast doubt on the value of using oxygen at all. Resuscitations are now started using room air, and we gradually increase the oxygen level only if there's no response.

By the early 1960s neonatal doctors had developed a range of techniques to save babies, but they were applied nowhere near as widely as they might have been. That changed dramatically after 1963 following the birth of Patrick Kennedy – the fourth child of US president John F Kennedy and Jacqueline Bouvier

Kennedy. Patrick was born five weeks early weighing 2110 grams, and died 39 hours later from respiratory distress syndrome (RDS) – a condition that was all too common at the time, where the lungs are immature so they can't inflate properly (the same condition that afflicted the baby boy I watched die in Rotorua Hospital as a trainee).

After such a high-profile death, the United States poured huge sums into the care of preterm infants and within a decade that started to take effect: the rate of RDS-related infant mortality in the US dropped dramatically in the early 1970s.

The rate would have dropped even more drastically if doctors in the US had kept a closer eye on what was happening on the other side of the world – down in New Zealand.

In 1967, Auckland obstetrician Graham Liggins was conducting experiments on sheep, looking into the role of the foetus in controlling the timing of its own birth. One experiment involved injecting ewes with the steroid hormone cortisol, bringing on an early labour. Liggins noticed that those cortisol-induced lambs seemed able to breathe far better than they should have for their gestational age; and after dissection he could see that their lungs were partly air-filled. In an inspired leap of reasoning, he figured that the cortisol must have accelerated the maturation of the foetus's lungs, and wondered whether the same process might work in humans.

Liggins and his colleague Ross Howie designed a trial where mothers going into premature labour were given cortisol injections. The results, published in 1972, were dramatic: cortisol injections led to a halving of death rates in preterm infants and a similar reduction in RDS. This was a game-changer, and led to swift improvements in neonatal survival in New Zealand. Incredibly, despite this clear evidence and the near-absence of side effects, the use of antenatal steroids didn't become routine in the US until the 1990s.

Since the 1970s there have been so many advances in neonatal medicine that it's impossible to list them all here. Few have had the transformative impact of Liggins and Howie's breakthrough, but step by step researchers have added strategies that improve babies' odds of surviving, and surviving without major disability. We have benefited from clever new drugs and new uses for old ones, from better methods for imaging and monitoring babies, from new blood transfusion techniques, from better ventilation systems and fancier incubators. We've steadily made changes to the human side of things, too: how we interact with parents and the kind of help we expect from them; how we gain consent for treatments and research trials.

In the march of progress, it is sometimes two steps forward and one step back. I mentioned the disastrous misuse of oxygen in the 1950s. We then learnt how to ventilate babies by inserting a breathing tube into their lungs. Later, when we realised that tube ventilation was causing scarring of the lungs, we moved to continuous positive airway pressure (CPAP) assistance – delivering air under pressure, using prongs up the nose, to keep the lungs inflated; the babies still regulate their own breathing. For a time, high-frequency oscillatory ventilation looked promising – this is where we jostle air/oxygen into the lungs rather than push it in under pressure. We still use it in certain situations, but recent studies have suggested CPAP is better.

Some important developments, such as the use of artificial surfactants, took a frustratingly long time to bed in. Healthy lungs are coated with a soapy substance called surfactant that helps each alveolus inflate like a tiny soap bubble. Usually, premature babies haven't yet produced enough surfactant of their own to breathe successfully. In 1959 American doctor John Clements started designing experimental synthetic surfactants that could be squirted directly into the lungs. It would be almost 30 years, though, before Japanese researchers showed that artificial surfactants were effective and safe in practice – at which point their use led to another jump in neonatal survival rates.

In New Zealand, Liggins' legacy of life-saving innovation continued, perhaps most notably with the work of Tania Gunn, Alistair Gunn and Peter Gluckman, who proved in the early 2000s that if a baby suffered brain damage during labour and delivery because of a lack of oxygen (known as perinatal asphyxia), some of this could be dramatically reduced by cooling the baby's head. Their research – which, like Liggins' research, began with experiments on sheep – was built in part on the observations of Norwegian researcher Marianne Thoresen, who noticed that during Norwegian winters children who fell through ice and 'drowned' for long periods in the frigid water below could be revived with little or no lasting brain damage. Cooling the brain appears to interrupt the usual process of apoptosis, where the death of cells from an initial injury inspires surrounding cells to undergo 'programmed cell death' – essentially a chain reaction of cell suicides. Cooling caps or body jackets like those trialled by the Gunn team are now standard equipment in neonatal wards for babies who have suffered asphyxia.

Some important changes are not technological – quite the opposite. In 1978 Colombian paediatrician Edgar Rey Sanabria was working in an NICU in Bogotá that was seriously short of staff and hi-tech equipment, so he began a regime where mothers spent as much time as possible holding their premature baby skin-to-skin on their chest and, where possible, breastfeeding.

This pragmatic, back-to-nature approach yielded great results, with the babies showing improvements in temperature management, heart rate, breathing, sleep and weight gain. Despite fears that the additional contact might increase rates of infection, that didn't happen. Sanabria's methods – known as 'kangaroo care' – are now used around the world.

This is one of the ways that parents have been welcomed back into the NICU, where they're encouraged to touch, feed and talk to their babies as much as possible without compromising care. While Stéphane Tarnier showed the world in 1880 that technology could do certain things better than nature, one of the successes of modern neonatology has been to acknowledge that the reverse is also true.

***

One of the awful things about the chest physiotherapy tragedy in the National Women's NICU was that this wasn't even a treatment we considered of huge importance. We barely even thought of it as a treatment; it was just a part of routine daily care, like suctioning saliva from a baby's mouth, or washing and turning the baby, or cleaning their incubator every few days. That was why it didn't even make it into the initial list of 50 possible risk factors in Harding's statistical analysis.

Chest physiotherapy was performed mostly on babies who were breathing with the help of tube ventilation. A tube down the windpipe all day means throat secretions can't be brought up in the usual way, leading to a higher risk of pneumonia. So in NICUs all over the world, staff found ways to loosen the buildup of mucus.

One technique was to place a buzzing electric toothbrush on the baby's chest. Another method was to put a small rubber cup on the chest and vibrate it gently four or five times a second with your hand, rather like a miniature sink-plunger. The point of the rubber cup was to ensure that the energy was dissipated across a wider area. After 10 minutes or so of light 'chest-tapping' the mucus would have loosened; then the mucus was suctioned out from the windpipe. There was no formal research to prove it worked but it made perfect sense, and it wasn't dissimilar to some of the techniques of 'chest physical therapy' used to greatly enhance and prolong the lives of cystic fibrosis sufferers. It became an established practice in NICUs around the world, but was not based on evidence.

Nowadays, if you were to introduce a new technique like this to an NICU, you would most likely do a pilot study of 50 or so babies and compare them with 50 untreated babies to see if the treated group improved faster, whether they were less susceptible to pneumonia, whether they had less chronic lung disease later, and so on. Back then, though, it was considered reasonable just to look around the world, see what other folk were doing and say, 'Well, we should probably do that too.'

What we now know is that in some instances of chest physiotherapy, especially if the treatment was vigorous or went on too long, the vibration of the chest may have caused brief spikes in blood pressure in the major blood vessels in the torso, and some of that pressure must have been transferred up into the cranial blood vessels, causing the devastating bleeds.

***

After Harding's phone conversation with Birmingham, and the immediate halt of further physiotherapy in our unit, we phoned the parents of the 13 babies affected as soon as possible and arranged for a consultant and a social worker to visit each of them. These were tough visits to make. For each visit we would ask the parents to sit down and we would then say: 'Look, we've got some news we want to share with you that is pretty serious and possibly very upsetting. We have recently discovered that those brain haemorrhages that your baby had may have been caused by the physiotherapy.' The parents I visited were shocked, though they seemed less angry than I might have expected. Often the anger came later, once they'd had a few days to absorb the news.

At the time, some media commentators suggested a cover-up was taking place, but this was the exact opposite of the truth. We communicated everything as quickly and openly as we could. We set up an 0800 phone number for our preterm parents to call. We informed NICU units around the world, put out a press release telling media what had happened and, in time, published a journal article with more details.

Because the injuries and deaths of the babies were the result of a medical mishap, families were compensated by the Accident Compensation Corporation (ACC). The ACC recommended a full ministerial inquiry that finally began five years later, in 1999, led by Helen Cull QC. It was nerve-racking having to get up and read out our statements to the inquiry in the manner of a witness at a criminal trial. We knew that if we were found in some way negligent, our careers were on the line. It was especially tough on the physiotherapists and nurses who had been taught how to use the technique and were only carrying out our instructions.

In work like this at the extremes of viability there will always be situations where we will make babies worse rather than better, and the experimental nature of much of what we do may even contribute to babies dying. As clinicians in charge of the babies' care, accepting that we are not always going to get it right is part and parcel of our job: if we can't wear that openly and honestly, we're in the wrong job.

We felt bad about what had happened, yet we all felt we had acted correctly given what we knew at the time. We had performed standard neonatal intensive care on vulnerable babies at the limits of viability. When we'd noticed a new problem we had investigated it, found the cause of the problem and addressed it, then we'd disclosed our findings openly and apologised to parents, while offering them support. If we were hung out to dry after having been so transparent, what message would that be sending to other NICUs, and to the medical profession in general, about how to deal with errors in the future?

As a team we were upset that the Birmingham hospital, when faced with almost exactly the same circumstances as us, had failed to sound the general alarm that might have pre-empted the problem at our unit and others. Birmingham hadn't even informed its parents about what had happened to the 15 or so babies hurt or killed by the brain bleeds; they'd simply stopped doing the physiotherapy. It would be ludicrous, we thought, if that became the model for how to behave, while we at National Women's were crucified for being honest and open.

Adding to the furore around this case were the echoes of the Cartwright Inquiry of 1988 which found that doctors at National Women's had behaved unethically while treating women with cervical cancer. A central issue there was that Herbert Green had enrolled his patients in a research programme without letting them know, and inadequate consent had been sought for various treatments and procedures. That inquiry's recommendations utterly transformed the relationship between doctors and patients in New Zealand, rewrote the ethical rules around consent and led to the formation of the Office of the Health and Disability Commissioner.

It was all too tempting for media to draw parallels between the Cartwright Inquiry and the Cull Inquiry 11 years later: was this the same hospital causing mayhem by once again playing fast and loose with issues of consent?

Ultimately, the Cull Inquiry found we had acted appropriately throughout, including around consent: a survey of all the level 3 NICUs in New Zealand and some in Australia and the United Kingdom confirmed that, like us, none of them had thought to ask for consent to use physiotherapy. It was a huge relief, with the inquiry complete, to have reached the end of a difficult time. It was, we thought, all over.

Except it wasn't quite. The following year two families lodged formal complaints with the Medical Council against Jane Harding, David Knight and myself. Similar complaints were made to the Nursing Council and Physiotherapists Board against individual nurses and physiotherapists.

For me, this was too much. We had devoted our careers to saving these vulnerable little babies. It was Harding who had laboured to identify the cause of this new problem when it arose. It was Knight who had walked into the ward and halted the physiotherapy. The nurses and physiotherapists had been doing their jobs and doing their best. In a moment of anger and frustration I told journalist Donna Chisholm, 'If this complaint doesn't go away I am giving up neonatology.' I felt uncomfortable criticising parents who I knew had already suffered terribly, but even 17 years after the fact, I stand by what I said to Chisholm: 'We are practising at the frontiers of medicine in neonatology; we are carrying out treatments today which are being carried out worldwide and people will look back in 10 years and say that wasn't the best way to do things. But that is what happens when you are trying to save babies who in nature should not be alive.'

The final wave of complaints were not upheld.

***

Sometimes a complaint made against a doctor will be fair. Sometimes it will not be fair but you can still understand the complainant's desire for someone to be held responsible for what has gone wrong. And sometimes you just shake your head at the cheek of it.

For a time, I was one of two paediatricians who looked after babies born to mothers who were addicted to opiates such as morphine, heroin or methadone. Opiates cross the placental barrier, so these babies are born addicted and, if left untreated, suffer withdrawal symptoms –

agitation and irritability, and they may also have fever, diarrhoea, trembling and fast breathing. To prevent this the babies are given small doses of morphine after birth, and are then safely weaned off the drug.

I was looking after one such baby whose mother had been in the methadone treatment programme during pregnancy when I noticed the treatment wasn't working. The baby – an otherwise healthy full-termer – was very unsettled, and wriggling so much that her elbows had rubbed raw. We kept increasing the morphine dose but nothing seemed to work.

The aha! moment arrived when the charge nurse happened to mention to me that there had been a problem with a nurse, who had since been dismissed, who had been caught stealing drugs from the drug cupboard.

I took the bottle of morphine we'd been using on the withdrawing baby and sent it to the pharmacy for analysis, where they found it was just water and contained no morphine at all. By then the baby had already weathered the withdrawal period, and though she'd obviously had a very unpleasant time of it, she wasn't going to suffer any lasting harm from having gone cold turkey.

I was feeling rather pleased with my successful sleuthing, and went to tell the mother what was going on: 'Look, we're very sorry, but we need to tell you that your baby was not being treated appropriately. Somebody had stolen the morphine so we were unknowingly giving her water.' She seemed to accept this, but later I learnt she had made a formal complaint about me.

I was asked to write a letter of response to the medical disciplinary committee. I could barely contain my indignation: I pointed out that it wasn't me who had taken opiates throughout a pregnancy, meaning my baby was forced to go through withdrawal. It wasn't me who'd stolen the morphine so the baby was being treated with water. I was the person who'd found the problem, rectified it and apologised to the mother on the hospital's behalf – so why was I the villain of the piece? The committee took my point and the problem melted away, but it had still been a nasty surprise.

***

Defending myself in front of a ministerial inquiry into chest physiotherapy, then fending off complaints to the Medical Council over the same issue, forced me to reflect on what this job meant to me and whether the rewards were worth the risks. I'm glad I was never put to the test on my threat to quit neonatology if we were found at fault: I would have missed it. I felt we were working under a cloud during those years, and it definitely took the shine off some of the everyday pleasures of helping vulnerable babies. But we learnt some valuable lessons.

Immediately after the inquiry's report, a working group was formed to see how we could improve consent processes in intensive care units, given that hundreds of different procedures are done daily and rules requiring written consents for each and every procedure would bring the unit to a grinding halt. The working group, composed of intensive care doctors and nurses, lawyers, lay representatives, ethicists and academics, helped us define more clearly which procedures could be covered with a quick chat at the time, which required more in-depth discussion (for example, something invasive like a lumbar puncture) and which needed full written consent (surgery).

Having to rethink and rework the issues of how consent works in a busy intensive care unit reminded me of the profound importance of the relationship between neonatologists and parents. If a parent is being told about a planned procedure on their child and objects, a discussion ensues and the reasons for doing the procedure are outlined. Once things have been explained it is unusual for the parents to then stop it from going ahead. The vast majority of the time, we clinicians see parents as our partners, and I believe that most of them feel the same way. Parents depend on us to look after their children but we absolutely need their involvement, too. We need their day-to-day support in doing our job in the ward. We need their consent and cooperation as we look after their child.

But also this: none of the extraordinary advances in neonatology over the past century that I've described would have been possible without the incredible generosity of the parents who allow their babies to participate in research trials. Most parents are keen to help. It's fortuitous, also, that babies involved in trials have been shown to do a little better, on average – probably because they're being monitored and measured more closely than others.

Babies from our NICU were involved in the groundbreaking work by the Gunns and Gluckman on the benefits of cooling a newborn's head. Christine McIntosh carried out a study into possible links between cot death (sudden infant death syndrome) and car seats: her study found that a simple foam-rubber insert could reduce risky drops in oxygen levels while a preterm baby was napping in a car seat.

In Auckland, Ed Mitchell led a hugely influential three-year study into cot death, which was one of the first studies to show that laying babies on their front or side to sleep was dangerous. With the introduction of the 'Back to Sleep' campaign there was a plunge in the rate of cot deaths – in New Zealand, rates reduced from more than four per 1000 live births in the 1980s to less than one per 1000 live births: over 3000 babies' lives were saved from 1990 to 2009. The same policy has since been introduced in other countries.

Meanwhile, researchers in neonatal wards worldwide are finding new ways to push back that margin between survival and death. That's a good-news story in many ways. But with each new intervention that's invented, we neonatologists are forced to confront afresh one of the fundamental questions of our trade. That question is not: 'Can we keep this child alive?', but 'Should we?'

CHAPTER 4

BABY L

The fundamental principle of medical ethics is 'first, do no harm'.

In early 2017, the parents of a baby boy in the United Kingdom launched an internet appeal. They were raising funds for an experimental treatment that they hoped might save their child from a lethal genetic disorder that had robbed him of muscle strength and was making him sicker by the day.

Doctors at London's Great Ormond Street Hospital had initially been willing to try the treatment on their patient, but when the boy's condition collapsed they told his parents the only sensible course was to turn off the life support and switch to palliative care – making the baby as comfortable as possible while letting him die naturally. The parents didn't agree.

That baby's name was Charlie Gard, and his story made headlines around the world.

For the doctors, the situation seemed clear: Charlie's mitochondrial disorder was destroying his brain and causing persistent seizures. He was deaf, his internal organs were failing and he could no longer breathe or move without assistance. Eventually, he would die. Yes, the hospital had equipment that could keep him alive for quite a while longer, but it was delaying the inevitable and Charlie was possibly suffering. The parents, meanwhile, still had faith in the experimental treatment. Eventually the hospital appealed to the British courts, asking for permission to withdraw life support without parental consent.

I had no involvement whatsoever in the case, but I couldn't help following the headlines closely, watching with concern as the case of poor little Charlie Gard became an international political football, kicked around by religious conservatives and political opportunists. The Vatican released a statement, and President Donald Trump and his ultraconservative deputy Mike Pence weighed in to support the parents, despite Charlie's hopeless prognosis. Activists from the pro-life movement painted the issue as a clash between medical authoritarian rule and parental rights. Some of America's less reputable media outlets promoted the lie that this was proof that under Britain's socialised health system, lifesaving treatment could be halted by the government when it got too expensive.

Doctors don't like taking parents to court for the right to let a baby die. I know this first-hand. The reason I couldn't take my eyes off the saga of Charlie Gard was because in 1999, at National Women's Hospital in Auckland, I had found myself caught up in a remarkably similar case.

***

'Baby L' was a lovely little girl who was born at National Women's in 1999, seven weeks premature. She looked normal for her gestational age, but it was immediately apparent that she wasn't breathing on her own and would need NICU help. She was a patient of my colleague

David Knight, and I was part of the wider team of consultants responsible for her care.

Over a couple of days, as we ruled out various possible causes for the breathing problems, it became obvious she had other problems, too. She appeared to be blind and deaf, and her facial muscles were paralysed.

Eventually, with the help of EEGs and MRIs and the expert opinion of a neurologist, we diagnosed two disorders: Moebius syndrome, where multiple cranial nerves have failed to develop, and Poland syndrome, where chest muscles are underdeveloped. Baby L would never see, speak, hear, eat or breathe unassisted. We suspected she was able to feel pain, but, if so, she wasn't able to communicate her distress because of the paralysed facial muscles.

With a diagnosis this devastating we don't rush things. It took a week or two to clarify absolutely that there was no way her condition could improve and that she would, sooner or later, die despite our best efforts. Then we began the difficult but inevitable conversation with her parents about the need to 'redirect care' away from the mechanical continuation of life we could offer on the unit. That's when it became complicated.

Her parents, devout Mormons, were unwilling to make a choice that would lead to the death of their child. Faced with an impossible situation, the hospital's ethics committee eventually applied to the High Court in Auckland to end the life support without their consent, on the grounds that further treatment was 'futile and therefore inhumane'. It was the first time such a request had ever been taken to a New Zealand court.

In a day-long hearing in front of two judges, Knight said that the treatment we were providing Baby L was only 'delaying her death and delaying it in a fairly unpleasant manner'. We asked for the baby to be made a ward of the state, which would give us the right to turn off the machines.

There was no animosity between the medical team and the parents. As Knight said in court, we had enormous respect for Baby L's mother and the care she had shown Baby L. He said: 'What makes us saddest is not that we are applying to the court, but that we are giving her the news that we don't think her baby can survive.'

This was an unprecedented situation, and there was huge media interest. Here was a beautiful-looking baby, and the hospital was telling her parents that she needed to die. The story drew some international attention as well – the BBC came to New Zealand to make a documentary about the case – but fortunately the coverage never reached the levels of rhetoric and hysteria that would be whipped up around the Charlie Gard case. I suppose that's partly because 20 years ago social media barely existed, so stories didn't go viral in quite the same way, but I suspect it was also because New Zealand media tend to be more level-headed than the worst of the British tabloids. Rather than stoking heated online arguments – and ignorant interjections from the likes of the US president – the case of Baby L stirred up a deeply empathetic reaction from the New Zealand public as they were given a glimpse into some of the ethical dilemmas that parents and staff routinely face in NICU wards.

The judges made Baby L a ward of state on a Thursday. Although it had taken a court's intervention to secure the cooperation of Baby L's parents, I had a strong sense that they were relieved by a ruling that took the decision out of their hands. They understood that their child was going to die soon, one way or another. It was just that they themselves couldn't bear to make the active choice that would hasten her death.

By the Saturday morning, with the full cooperation of the parents, we had made arrangements for Baby L to go home for the first time in her life, with a portable incubator and ventilator. Friends and extended family gathered for a 30-minute prayer service and kissed the baby goodbye. I wasn't there, but David Knight and a number of Baby L's NICU nurses were, as well as a newspaper journalist who would describe the scene in the next day's paper.

At 10am, Baby L's mother held her baby in her arms as one of the nurses removed the breathing tube and the portable ventilator was turned off. Her mother then carried her into the back garden, and a couple of minutes later Baby L died. She was nine weeks old.

Baby L's death had been handled with dignity and respect. Our ability to sustain life a little longer hadn't overruled the stronger moral imperative to let nature take its course when there was no hope, and when a baby was suffering because of our efforts to keep her alive.

***

After a complex legal battle, Charlie Gard's life support was ended on 27 July 2017. He died the next day, just short of one year old.

There were important differences between the circumstances of Charlie Gard in 2017 and Baby L in 1999, but the underlying question was the same: When all prospect of a meaningful life for a sick baby is gone, there is no hope of recovery and they may be suffering pain, but you have the technical ability to keep them alive for just a little longer, should you do so?

For me, the answer to this is a resounding 'no'. To think otherwise is to fall prey to the 'technological imperative' – the belief that if we *have* the technology we *must use* the technology. It's an attitude that is regrettably common in medicine in the United States but has, thankfully, mostly failed to take hold in New Zealand.

In clearcut cases like those of Baby L and Charlie Gard, the answer can seem easy. Yet a broader – and much trickier – version of this question is being addressed every day in neonatal wards all over the world: How do we know if the time has come to stop trying to keep this baby alive, and instead to help him or her die in the best possible way?

We cannot and should not save the life of every baby, yet trying to figure out which life is worth saving and which life is not is one of our hardest tasks. No one feels proud to have saved the life of a baby who faces a miserable future of constant suffering. Equally, no one feels proud about failing to offer lifesaving intensive care to an infant who might have survived and gone on to live a fulfilling life.

What makes these decisions even harder is that the long-term 'value' of a life is all but uncountable, and it depends very heavily on who's doing the counting. Studies of extremely preterm infants who have reached their late teens and early twenties show that these young people value their own lives just as highly as their peers who were born full-term, and this holds true regardless of whether they are living with a lasting disability or not.

Another issue – which we never discuss with parents, but which lurks beneath the surface of any conversation about the ethics of intensive care – is one of cost. We naturally want as many resources for our department as we can get, but in a state-funded healthcare system facing limitless demands, what might be done elsewhere with the $3000 a day that it costs for us to keep a baby alive?

When pushed on this, as I was recently in conversation with a taxi driver who reckoned saving extremely preterm babies was an unnecessary drain on the economy. I happily argued that neonatal care offers pretty good value for money. The cost of four or five months in NICU is still less than a kidney transplant or a heart bypass once you take into account the number of productive years that it offers to the patient: a lifetime in the case of the preterm baby versus a decade or so in the case of a 75-year-old cardiac patient.

A parent's perspective is very different from that of medical staff, and staff themselves may disagree. We consultants oversee a baby's treatment based on three short ward visits a day, but nurses provide the minute-by-minute care over eight- or 12-hour shifts, so they are the ones who are confronted with a baby's pain and discomfort when being subjected to frequent blood tests and constant suctioning of the mouth, or recovering from emergency surgery. Their awareness of a baby's suffering is more intimate and acute. More than once I have been collared by a nurse demanding to know why we are continuing heroic measures to keep a baby alive: 'If you can't see a future for this baby then why are you carrying on? You wouldn't do this to your pet!'

Our decisions are fallible, and sometimes a baby will remind us of that in the loveliest way possible. Some years ago, the parents of a baby of 24 weeks' gestation whose delivery was imminent told us they didn't want any intensive care at all once the child had arrived. They'd read widely about extreme prematurity and didn't want to put the baby, or themselves, through it all. Twenty-four weeks is on the very margin of survivability, and although these days we offer intensive care to babies as early as 23 weeks if parents want it, we agreed this was a very reasonable decision for them to make. (For 25-weekers of a good size we are more insistent on offering care, as the odds of a good outcome are much higher.)

I checked with the mother again during labour and she was adamant they wanted no intervention. After the birth the baby girl was placed on her chest so they could spend her final hours cuddling skin-to-skin.

Six hours later I was called back to talk to the puzzled parents. Their daughter was breathing surprisingly well and was quite pink. We made a joint decision to institute intensive care with the proviso that, if things went badly, we could still abandon that course. We wrapped the baby in a warm blanket and her father carried her up to the NICU, surprising the nurses who were more used to 24-weekers arriving in a transport incubator with bells and whistles blasting. Once there, she was slotted in to the usual intensive-care scenario: incubator, ventilation, oxygen, intravenous lines. She did very well and was discharged home a few months later, breastfeeding and thriving. The last time I heard from the parents she was a happy and healthy 10-year-old, and her parents love her to bits.

***

In the past half-century the relationship between patient and doctor has changed profoundly – mostly for the better. Doctors are no longer godlike figures whose word must not be questioned. Patients' informed consent must be obtained before procedures are carried out, except in acute life-saving emergencies. 'Paternalism' is a dirty word; it has been replaced by consumer empowerment. In a health system like New Zealand's where patients aren't directly confronted with the cost of various treatments, there is also a tendency among doctors to say: 'These are all the treatment options – which one would you like?'

In neonatal care, though, I believe there is still a strong case for being directive in supporting parental decisions. Parents are trying to make life-and-death decisions about their precious new baby while under extreme emotional pressure – and often after days without sleep. No one sets out to be the parent of a preterm infant, and few people are well equipped to understand every nuance of a fast-changing and medically complex situation. So doctors have to shoulder some of that responsibility and give parents a firm nudge in the right direction. We know we won't always get it right, but we have to trust our decades of experience.

I will say to parents: 'We can keep almost everybody alive these days, but I don't think keeping a baby alive for the sake of it is justifiable. There is a difference between being alive, and having a life.'

And sometimes, as hard as it may seem, I will say: 'No, I'm afraid we're not going to offer this treatment.'

These are tough messages, but if honesty and transparency are balanced with kindness and compassion, we can guide parents towards the best option, even when it runs counter to their initial instincts. The process is always one of collaboration between the families and the medical and nursing staff, and involves many difficult conversations over several days. Very occasionally, when we reach an impasse, we will also involve the hospital ethics committee.

Sometimes the roles are reversed and it's the doctor fighting for a baby after a parent wants to give up. I'll never forget attending the delivery of a baby whose parents had decided not to have the amniocentesis test for trisomy 21 during the pregnancy, in part because they had a much-loved relative with Down syndrome. It looked to me, once the baby was born, as if he probably did have Down syndrome. Not only that, he had other complications that had left him hugely bloated with fluid and needing intensive breathing support.

I told the new parents I suspected Down syndrome, and the mother said: 'Please, I don't want you to resuscitate this baby.'

'I don't think we can do that,' I answered. 'I don't have enough information to make a decision as important as that.'

The mother was adamant she didn't want the baby, so while the nurse practitioner continued the resuscitation I quickly phoned a colleague. I rattled off the details and asked if he thought I should carry on. He agreed that given the likelihood of an eventual good outcome, I was indeed ethically obliged to carry on. I returned to the mother and said, 'I'm sorry, but I have to try.'

The kicker came a couple of years later when the mother brought her son in for a follow-up appointment. I said, 'Do you remember what you said when this baby was born?' She replied, 'I'll tell you what. If you had *not* resuscitated him I would have taken you to the cleaners.' I've no idea if that's truly what she would have done, but what I could see for certain was that she loved that child very much.

When a baby is really struggling and sick, it's not unheard of for a parent to discreetly ask me if there isn't something we could do to hasten what looks like an inevitable death.

I can see why they ask, and one might argue that there is no logical difference between *letting* a baby die by taking it off life support and *making* a baby die with, say, a lethal injection. But from a medical and moral perspective, that difference is enormous and insurmountable. We can never cross that line into euthanasia, because that is not what we are here to do. The fundamental principle of medical ethics is 'first, do no harm'.

There is one area that from the outside might appear grey: giving an opiate such as morphine when a baby is in great pain, with the knowledge that the painkiller may hasten death because it suppresses respiration. But when you look closely, even this grey resolves to a clearcut black and white: the drug is being used only for pain relief, and the risk to respiration is a side effect that we have learnt to live with.

***

It is never easy to start the conversation with a parent about the possibility of 'allowing a natural death', or 'redirecting' the care of their baby. (We prefer the term 'redirect' to 'withdraw' because switching to end-of-life care means an *increase* in the resources and nursing support devoted to a baby from then until death.)

In this job, finding the path to a good death is equally as important as saving a life. As well as a clinical change of focus, this is a time to consider what memories a family will want to take away. That might mean taking photos, foot and hand imprints or a lock of hair; or a parent changing a nappy for the first time because the baby has previously been too sick even to touch; or inviting friends or family to pay a visit.

We always arrange follow-up interviews about six weeks after a baby's death. I'm struck by how positive parents' memories of the day are. For many, this will have been the first time they really *saw* their baby with all the tubes and tapes and needles removed. Whether it's in the unit or at home, like Baby L, the baby will usually spend their final moments in a parent's arms rather than in an incubator. Some parents remember it as a special day of a very difficult period in their lives.

On a couple of occasions I've treated babies who were born entirely without brain tissue, but with enough brainstem function that they could breathe unaided. Theoretically, such a child could be kept alive indefinitely with tube feeding, in a sort of perpetual half-life, but another approach is to allow nature to take its course by sending the baby home with support from a homecare nurse, and feeding the baby when they're hungry, providing medicine for any discomfort and letting them die in their own time.

I once helped the parents of a child with a missing heart ventricle by arranging 'comfort and support' palliative care at home, after they decided they didn't want us to attempt a series of complex and highly risky operations. Some days later, the parents asked me to come and visit: they weren't sure if their baby had died. When I arrived she wasn't quite there yet, so I said, 'We'll just sit here for a while and see what happens. We're not going to do anything.' And the child eventually slipped away. It was a curiously beautiful moment.

***

In 1985, faced with a three-month gap between two jobs, I left my wife Ann and our two toddlers in Auckland and spent those months at an American hospital in Khamis Mushayt in Saudi Arabia.

The work was similar to what I'd been doing in Auckland, but the patients were not. King Faisal Hospital was a women's and children's hospital for the Saudi military, and money was not in short supply. On one occasion I escorted a newborn baby who needed an emergency surgery that could only be performed in the port city of Jeddah. We took the ambulance out to the airfield and boarded a Lear jet. As we took off, I watched in awe as the mountains around us turned to pink and purple in the dusk.

The hospital itself was heavily guarded; no local men were allowed inside. There were spacious courtyards with oleander, hibiscus, tea roses and brightly coloured impatiens. A common sight was several women crouching around a coffee pot on the ground, enjoying each other's company and dishes of fresh dates.

I soon realised I would need to change my assumptions about how women operated in this society that was outwardly so patriarchal. With no Muslim men about, the extreme rules around modesty and covering oneself didn't apply. The black headgear was discarded back in the wards and the women were beautifully made-up and wearing masses of jewellery. On the first day on the neonatal unit I was explaining to a young mother about her premature baby's likely progress and asked whether she was intending to breastfeed. I was shocked when she opened her blouse and showed me her breast and said, 'See, I don't have any milk.'

At times, my doctoring style was lost in the translation between English and Arabic. On one occasion I asked the interpreter, a Lebanese man, to tell a mother that her child was beautiful. He said nothing to her, and when I asked him why later he shrugged and said, 'She doesn't need to know that.'

In the obstetric hospital the rate of births by caesarean section was 2.5 per cent, compared with well over 20 per cent in New Zealand at that time. The difference was partly that most of the women were delivering their sixth or seventh child, but I also wondered whether the local practice of squatting rather than sitting might have stretched and toned their pelvic floor muscles to facilitate delivery.

That said, one time when it was thought a caesarean was needed – an obstructed labour with foetal distress – the father refused to give consent for surgery and the mother laboured on for another 24 hours and eventually, to my surprise, delivered the baby normally.

Being in Saudi was a fascinating opportunity to observe the universality of human qualities – kindness, warmth, good humour, tenderness towards children. I also noticed some real cultural differences, however. In particular, there was a pragmatism around infant mortality that I'd seldom encountered in the United Kingdom or in New Zealand – perhaps because families were so large.

More than once, when a woman had delivered prematurely and we had the baby in the incubator, she would head home, telling us to ring when the baby was fit to come home – and there would be no visits during the several months until the baby was ready.

Once, when a premature baby was dying, I tried to comfort the father. I said, 'I'm really sorry. It's so sad. This baby has come too early and we aren't going to be able to save him.' The father put his arm around me and said, 'Don't worry, doctor. Don't be upset. This is Allah's will and it will be all right. There will be more children to come.' I almost felt like I needed to keep on feeling upset because *someone* had to be sad about the death of this baby.

***

When tragedy is part of your daily routine you need to be ready for it, but you can't just turn off the emotional tap. I don't think I have hardened over the years on the neonatal ward, but nor have I become more soppy and emotional. Rather, I have come to accept that things will still touch me when I don't expect them to, and that I will sometimes be overcome with sadness or anger, or both.

The fact that a baby has died may not affect me deeply, especially where death has seemed like the best of the possible outcomes. What always does move me, though, is the parents' own grief and distress, particularly when I see a father in tears – perhaps because it's so much harder for men, especially New Zealand men, to openly express emotion.

I sometimes cry in front of parents, and from a professional perspective that's not necessarily a bad thing. Parents can take comfort from knowing that you share some of their pain, and it's valuable for junior staff too to see that even folk like me who've been doing this for decades are still affected. We have a responsibility to mentor junior staff through emotionally tough situations.

That said, it's no good if parents end up comforting me rather than experiencing their own grief, so I try to make sure I'm not falling apart when parents really need my confidence and support. Like anyone, I'm more emotionally vulnerable when tired or sleep-deprived, so there have been times at the end of a long shift when I've sloped off to a corner for a quick private weep, rather than do it in front of parents.

A baby's death is especially tough on the nurses who have developed an intimate connection through hour-by-hour care. We encourage the nurses who were closest to a baby to go to the funeral. I don't get to every funeral – far from it – but when I do I can usually keep myself together until the music begins. When they start singing 'The Lord's My Shepherd', I turn to jelly.

CHAPTER 5

AUTISM, ADHD AND OTHER ADVENTURES

One of my first goals after diagnosis was to help parents overcome their own doom and gloom about the obstacles ahead.

It had been a perfect Boxing Day at our tennis club, an afternoon of mixed doubles and good food and splashing about in the swimming pool – though due to our paranoia around water, Ann and I agreed that if one of us was swinging a racquet, the other had to sit out to keep an eye on our three sons, especially our youngest, Tom, who at two and a half was not an enthusiastic swimmer.

Now, though, it was time to head home. We were heading out the gate when a woman rushed past us on the path, pausing only to ask if we knew where to find a phonebox.

It was at that moment that I noticed Tom wasn't with us. I headed back to see what had waylaid him, and noticed a small huddle at the poolside and someone performing a resuscitation. I assumed it was a heart attack, but as I got closer I realised it was a child – then I recognised the blue T-shirt. It was Tom.

I rushed forward, heart pounding, and at that moment Tom sat up and coughed out a surprising amount of water and barbecued sausage. As he was loaded onto the ambulance stretcher a few minutes later, he said: 'Dad, I don't want to go to bed.' This made me suspect he was probably going to be OK, but we headed to hospital for an assessment anyway.

Later we figured out what must have happened. After a day of watching our boy like a hawk, we hadn't been looking behind us as we filed past the pool on our way out, and Tom must have tripped, fallen in and sunk straight to the bottom. A minute or two later a 12-year-old girl said: 'Mum, I think there's a baby at the bottom of the pool.' Her mother glanced over and said 'No, I think that's just a towel.' Then she took another look, and dived in fully dressed.

For years afterwards I would wake most mornings with a jolt of horror at the realisation of how close we had come to losing our child. Later still, I realised it was another of the small ways that my own experience as a parent helped inform my work as a paediatrician.

Ann, in particular, was always super-vigilant around water, to the extent that when we went to the beach she'd covertly unpack my novel before we left so I could give my full attention to scanning the shallows for sharks and drowning children. If *we* could come that close to disaster, who was I to judge a parent whose child needed my help after darting in front of a car, or swallowing poison while unsupervised, or falling out of a tree? Bad things happen, and there but for the grace of God go I.

***

I was heading towards a career in paediatrics by my mid twenties, and didn't have my first child until I was in my mid thirties. During that decade, if you'd asked my opinion I'd have sworn that you didn't need to have children of your own to be a good paediatrician. The notion seemed mildly insulting, like saying you couldn't be a good psychiatrist unless you'd personally experienced psychiatric illness. I'd done my study. I'd read everything. I liked children. I had friends with children and could see what it was like to be a parent. That was enough, surely.

In a way, that's what I still believe. But there's no doubt that having children changed me professionally, for better and for worse. I found, for instance, that if I was looking after a dying or suffering child who was close in age to one of my own, I would be much more emotionally sensitive, which at times probably affected my judgement.

But I think such negatives were outweighed by a big positive – an increase in the empathy I felt for parents, and not only because of major events such as Tom's near-drowning. I think it's hard, for example, unless you've been a parent yourself, to understand the complex parental urge to throttle your much-loved child. When your own child is driving you insane, the idea of giving them a good slap is horribly appealing, even if it runs counter to your views about corporal punishment. And until you've been there yourself it can be hard to appreciate that kind of nuance.

The question has a flipside, of course: Does being a paediatrician make you a better *parent?* On this I'd say the jury is out. Children of medical professionals reputedly suffer from one of two curses: the parent who underdiagnoses every sniffle or ache because it seems trivial compared to the ghastly things they've seen at work; or the parent who overdiagnoses every sniffle or ache because it resembles a ghastly thing they've seen at work.

I've been guilty of both failings. My children know it's no use telling their dad when they are unwell, as he takes no notice. Son Joe returned from a Fiji surfing holiday with a flu-like illness, as had several of his friends. I said, 'We all get flu. Get over it.' It wasn't until I saw him stumbling and tripping like he was drunk that I realised it might be more serious: in the end he tested positive for dengue fever.

Conversely, when one of my boys had mumps (this was pre-measles immunisation) he became quite irritable and complained of headaches, and I convinced myself he had encephalitis, a dangerous but rare complication. Fortunately he got over it quickly, and so did I.

I tend to catastrophise my own health as well: every headache is a brain tumour; every time I forget a word I'm convinced that I have Alzheimer's. Once, when I had some numbness in my arm, I decided I had a spinal nerve tumour. I was sitting on the back steps thinking about the music I wanted for my funeral when I noticed the telltale rash and realised I had shingles.

***

Until very recently, on top of my neonatal hospital duties I used to work another 15 or so hours a week in private paediatric practice where my patients ranged from newborn to late teens (including some children I'd first encountered in hospital). Occasionally, a lesson I'd learnt from my own children proved professionally useful.

I remember a case where a 10-year-old boy came in with a cough that had persisted for six months. He'd had every imaginable examination – X-rays, asthma investigations, various treatment trials – but there was no obvious physical cause. The coughing continued unabated as he sat in my consulting room – more than a little annoyingly.

Some months earlier one of my own boys had had a similar cough. In his case I did no formal medical tests, as I doubted there was a serious physical cause (or perhaps I was being an underdiagnosing parent–doctor again). In any case, Ann and I had just ignored our son's cough and starved of attention it simply stopped in a matter of days.

I asked this 10-year-old to step out of my office for a moment while I chatted to his parents. I then asked them if they'd consent to me trying a simple behavioural modification. They told me to go for it. They were getting so desperate I suspect they'd have consented to the casting out of demons if I'd suggested it.

I called their son back in and talked directly to him. I pointed out that he was already missing lessons at school because he was being sent home sick, and that eventually he would start to lose friends because his cough was so annoying. I said I was confident he could take control of it himself: 'If you feel you're going to cough, try holding it back and don't do it, and in time it will get easier.' In short, I told him to stop.

That was a Thursday. On the Monday I rang his mother and asked how he was going. She said he hadn't coughed once since they'd left my office. It had been a sort of tic, which probably started with a cold and an itchy throat but then took on a life of its own. He was a perfectly well-adjusted normal kid, with well-adjusted parents, but at a subconscious level he was benefiting from all the attention and became trapped in a sort of psychological-meets-physical loop.

Some years later I saw a similar case of a girl who'd suffered chronic abdominal pain and gone through months of fruitless tests. She had come into the office crying and wailing very loudly – so much so that I had left my room to see whether she needed urgent help. As with the coughing boy, knowing that other specialists had already ruled out the likely physical causes gave me confidence to take a psychological tack without fearing I was overlooking something serious. I sat with the girl and told her she had the power to fix this herself. Her parents later reported that the pain had gone for good before they'd even reached home.

Once my own children became adolescents I found the firsthand experience of how teens behave very useful. Adolescence is a time of risk-taking, spending time with peers, sleeping a lot, and ignoring parents (though a few years later, as parents, you'll realise they were taking in more of what you were saying than it appeared).

So when an anxious parent said something like 'my son is sneaking out to parties instead of going to the library', I became increasingly confident in my soothing responses. Sometimes I wasn't sure whether I was using my medical training to help parents understand their teen, or relying on my own experiences.

I loved the broader perspective general paediatric work gave, and over the decades I saw nearly every imaginable condition I'd learnt about during training. I encountered brain tumours and metabolic disorders, injuries and infectious diseases, development problems and psychiatric disorders, babies with colic and teenagers with behavioural problems.

Like most doctors, I would get asked for ad hoc medical advice in social situations. Generally I'm happy to help, as long as I'm not expected to produce a definitive diagnosis and treatment plan while still holding my glass of pinot noir, and as long as the conversation can eventually move on to books, or independent films, or the rugby, or my garden. Occasionally media call me, too, asking for comment or advice on a newsworthy aspect of paediatrics. Certain topics come up time and again, so in the following sections I'm going to briefly touch on a few areas of paediatrics that might prove useful for parents who have concerns about their own children.

AUTISM SPECTRUM DISORDER/ASPERGER'S

'Tell me, what colour are my eyes?'

Here's how the consultation might go: A family arrives with their child, who is around three or four years old. The parents come in and say hello and we shake hands, but the child barely seems to notice I'm there, instead wandering around inspecting the room. He's not shy or embarrassed, either; no clinging to a parent for security. When I try to engage him – perhaps suggesting he come and sit on his mother's knee – he acts as if I've not even spoken. When the father says, 'Now, Jack, say hello to Dr Rowley,' it's the same – no reaction.

The parents are about to tell me more about their child and how he never listens and seems much naughtier than his peers, or how his language is behind his classmates' and he has few or no friends, or about their struggles to get him into the car when they leave anywhere, or his fussiness about the placement of food on his dinner plate, or his sensitivity to loud noises, or his constant lining up of his toy cars, or his repetitive flicking of switches. But before they've even opened their mouths, I've got a fair idea of what we face here, based purely on that first minute or two of the child's behaviour.

This is a child with autism spectrum disorder (ASD). The good news is that the future may not be as gloomy as the parents fear.

WHAT IS ASD?

Most likely, autism has been around as long as humans have existed, but it only began to be diagnosed from the 1940s when Leo Kanner in the US and Hans Asperger in Germany described children with characteristically withdrawn modes of behaviour, which were initially blamed on parenting styles. By the 1960s, though, researchers started to argue that there was something biologically different in the brains of autistic children.

As the name implies, the severity of ASD varies widely, but the clinical definition is pretty simple, with three main characteristics: impaired communication and delayed speech; inability to make normal social contact; and repetitive 'stereotypic' behaviours (such as rocking back and forth, flapping hands or flicking switches on and off). It appears to be the result of aberrant brain development that only becomes obvious from the age of 18 months or so, although it's very likely that the differences were already in play much earlier than that. The underlying cause, however, is still not clear.

Asperger originally described children with autistic features as having an extreme case of 'maleness'. They were more likely than their peers to 'systematise', and less interested in human relationships – the same differences that can be observed, on average, between boys and girls. (Studies have shown that even newborn boys and girls differ in this way: the girls spend relatively more time looking at faces and the boys looking at puzzles when they are put in front of them.)

Boys are between four and 15 times more likely to have autism than girls, depending on which data you look at. One intriguing study by British autism researcher Simon Baron-Cohen found an association between high levels of testosterone in a baby's amniotic fluid and subsequent development of autism. There are also associations with paternal age (the older the father, the more likely is autism in the child), and autistic traits can run in families, suggesting a strong genetic component. There is also a statistical association between babies being born preterm and being autistic.

Baron-Cohen has floated the theory that modern courting patterns, where workmates with the same intellectual propensities end up marrying each other, may explain the hotspots of autism in places such as San Francisco's Silicon Valley. He says when people in 'geeky', systematising careers such as computer engineering raise families together, their kids are getting a double dose of their parents' autistic traits.

The other thing keeping autism researchers awake at night is the question of why autism rates are currently soaring in the developed world. At medical school I learnt that autism affected around four or five in every 10,000 people. Today, that figure is closer to one in 100. Some of that change can be accounted for by 'diagnostic shift' (ie, we're looking for and identifying them more) – but certainly not all of it.

The one theory about autism we can safely ignore is the fraudulent research published by Andrew Wakefield in the United Kingdom, who suggested a link between autism and the childhood MMR (measles, mumps and rubella) vaccine. Irresponsible reporting of his wild claims led to a sharp drop in immunisation rates in the United Kingdom and worldwide, including in New Zealand. This, in turn, led to epidemics and dozens of totally avoidable deaths from diseases we had effectively conquered in most developed nations long ago.

Part of the appeal of this hoax theory was that the MMR vaccine was given to children at around 15 to 18 months of age – roughly the same time as autism symptoms start to reveal themselves. To this day I still encounter people who ask if MMR has anything to do with their child's autism, and I have to bite my tongue before politely stating that it's out of the question.

Some years ago I saw a child who had looked perfectly fine but then had seemingly abruptly displayed autistic traits right after his 18-month vaccination. It was fascinating, though, to talk to his parents after the arrival of their next child. Compared to their first, the second child was far more cheerful and engaging from very early on, and demonstrated a strong sense of humour and good social skills. The parents realised that their first child's 'normal' behaviour before he'd had his MMR jab had contained clear harbingers of the autism diagnosis.

One new and fascinating avenue of autism research concerns the 'microbiome' – the bacteria that live in harmony on and around us. The gut microbiome is in constant 'conversation' with the developing brain, sending and receiving messages at cellular and chemical levels. We acquire our gut microbiome from our mother as we come through the birth canal, but with caesarean deliveries now more common, and antibiotics frequently prescribed, we upset and change our bacterial flora. Although it is unlikely that alterations in our microbiome would affect our brain chemistry in such a way, it is interesting to speculate on it.

HOW WILL I KNOW IF MY CHILD HAS ASD?

The average baby will have figured out how to giggle by six to 10 weeks, and by three months will typically react with delight when a familiar face comes near.

If your baby's eye contact and tendency to giggle seem way behind their peers', don't worry too much, as babies do develop at different rates and there are numerous reasons other than autism why your child isn't making eye contact. But if you're worried, there's no harm in having a chat with your GP.

It's not until 18 to 24 months, though, that most parents really notice that their child seems a bit different. As well as repetitive behaviours and avoiding eye contact, an autistic child will miss social cues – they may not respond to their name or wave goodbye, or follow objects with their eyes when they're pointed out.

At later ages the behaviours are much the same but the consequences become more troubling – especially isolation from peers. It's hard to make a friend when you can't quite tell if the expression on your classmate's face is excitement, misery, boredom or anger. (Funnily enough, I've noticed children with ASD tend to be especially fond of the *Thomas the Tank Engine* stories and animation, which I suspect is partly because of the broad, unambiguous smiles and frowns of each train character.)

Many children with ASD weren't brought to me for a consultation until they were three or four, and that would be because their parents had been told by daycare or preschool staff that their child was having trouble with socialising and it might be worth a check-up. And if it wasn't spotted at daycare, it would almost certainly be spotted at school.

OK, MY CHILD DEFINITELY HAS ASD. WHAT NOW?

In private practice I tended to see children at the moderate end of the spectrum, including some with the relatively mild form known as Asperger's syndrome. One of my first goals after diagnosis was to help parents overcome their own doom and gloom about the obstacles ahead. There are no miracle cures for autism, but some relatively small steps can make a big difference. I generally gave parents three pieces of advice:

- You have a child who is quirky rather than naughty, interesting rather than weird, and who may even have some hidden talents – and these are all things to celebrate.
- Mild to moderate autism is a lifelong condition that can be managed – like diabetes or asthma – only instead of insulin or an inhaler

the treatment is regular, deliberate doses of socialisation.
- There are certain things your child will never find easy, so you will have to accommodate them and not the other way round.

A solo mother brought in her seven-year-old daughter who had ASD and was 'unmanageable'. She was refusing to get dressed for school, refusing to leave the house, refusing to respond when spoken to, and being rude to teachers and other adults, which the mother found mortifying. I sat down with the girl and asked her what was going on. Her answers were unusual yet cogent: the reason she had ignored her mother when she called her, for instance, was that she had been dressing her dolls, which was much more important than whatever her mother wanted.

After a fairly long chat, I told the mother that she had a smart, terrific – and quirky – child, and that if she stepped back from noticing every little failing those qualities might become more obvious. When we caught up again six months later, the mother said the household was transformed. In part that was because the girl was maturing, but it was also because the mother had eased off the constant tellings-off. She had gone looking for the good in her ASD child, and funnily enough she'd found it.

One of the clichés around ASD is that of the person who has socially crippling autistic traits alongside an extraordinary talent, like the prodigious counting skills of Dustin Hoffman's character in *Rain Man*. Such 'savants' certainly exist, but they're rare. In reality children with ASD have intelligence across a wide range, both below and above average. Still, it's not uncommon for someone with mild to moderate ASD to have one area that really stands out compared with their difficulties with socialising and language – mental arithmetic, say, or memorising pieces of music.

I have a colleague – a highly qualified paediatrician who is brilliant with computers and data analysis – who has come to realise that he lies somewhere at the mild end of the autistic spectrum. For those parts of the job that require a logical brain he's at a distinct advantage compared with me, and in those parts of the job that require empathy and social skills he has systematically applied his formidable intellect and figured out the most appropriate and effective ways to behave. He is kind with babies and wonderfully patient with parents, but those skills have grown out of careful observation and inquiry rather than instinct.

Fortunately the authentic, unpractised version of this lovely man is still just below the surface. For example, when he and his wife are over, he might pick up a book and start reading in the middle of a conversation. Like I said, you've got to find the quirks and enjoy them.

The best daily medicine for a child with mild to moderate ASD is socialisation. Skills such as meeting someone's eye or remembering to say 'hello', 'goodbye', 'please' and 'thank you' can be taught by rote, removing the need to rely on instincts that aren't there. (In a young child, I might trick them into initial eye contact by asking them to tell me what colour my eyes are.)

It's vital, though, that you never slip into stereotypical staunch Kiwi mode and tell a child with ASD to 'harden up'. That won't work. A social situation that might leave you feeling a little shy can be overwhelming to the point of trauma for an autistic child, so activities with large groups are seldom wise. Loud noises and other stimuli that you might find annoying, they can find physically painful.

As their parents soon learn, children with ASD like routine. An unannounced deviation from, say, the usual route to school can throw them out for the rest of the day. If change is coming, give them lots of warning that it's coming so they have time to get ready. And from quite a young age, there's a good chance that they'll remember precisely the route you took last time, even if it was six months earlier.

IF THERE'S NO CURE, IS A DIAGNOSIS EVEN USEFUL?

Not necessarily, though a formal diagnosis is extremely helpful if a child really needs a teacher aide or specialist education help, because the right label opens the doors to state funding.

Some parents find a diagnosis a huge relief: they realise they're not the only one struggling with their child's behaviour, and that there are some sensible steps they can take. Others, especially those whose child has only mild symptoms, would rather not have the label, and I'm happy to say to them, 'That's fine. Forget the label and focus on how best to help your special child navigate their way through life.'

ISN'T THERE A PILL OR SOMETHING YOU CAN PRESCRIBE?

Not really. Some people with ASD suffer crippling anxiety, and anxiolytic drugs that reduce anxiety levels, similar to Prozac, can help them manage that – but an effective drug-based treatment for ASD itself has yet to be found.

The situation gets more complicated in a child who, in addition to ASD, has attention deficit and hyperactivity disorder (ADHD). In this case, ADHD drugs such as Ritalin can be effective, but getting the prescription right isn't easy as the ADHD drugs can make ASD worse.

When parents get desperate they start looking around for other causes and cures, but I'm afraid there is very little good evidence for any of them. Diet hasn't been shown to make any difference. Acupuncture also hasn't been shown to work, and good luck with getting a needle into a child, anyway. With regard to omega-3 and omega-6 fatty acids, I would say 'watch this space'. The idea that they might improve brain function is plausible at a biological level, but there's no good research that proves they help with autism, and a recent New Zealand study carefully done as part of a PhD thesis and subsequently published in *Scientific Reports* found that many such oils sold in stores were rancid and thus potentially toxic rather than therapeutic.

What I do advise, though, is for parents to be rigorous in controlling their ASD child's access to screens. Autistic kids are often obsessively attracted to TVs, computer games, YouTube videos and the like. This is unhealthy for all the usual reasons, including lack of exercise and eating habits, but what concerns me most with regard to autism is what screens do to a child's socialisation. If you're watching a TV you're having zero interaction with the other side of the screen – yet social interaction is the very thing that autistic children need in higher doses than the average child.

One hunch I have, which seems to be supported by research studies with small sample sizes, is that autistic children benefit from hearing and making music, especially singing. Autism involves impairment of language and communication, but when you're singing you're recruiting parts of the brain that aren't usually used for making words.

ATTENTION DEFICIT AND HYPERACTIVITY DISORDER

'Oh, but his father was just the same!'

When I was at medical school in the early 1970s, attention deficit and hyperactivity disorder (ADHD) was an exotic diagnosis from the United States that wasn't even on the radar of doctors in Australasia or the United Kingdom. But 15 years later when I saw my first ADHD patient, there was no mistaking it.

The seven-year-old boy couldn't keep still – he was moving around in his chair, darting over to the toy box and pulling everything out, back to his seat, more fidgeting. Within minutes the room looked like a tornado had been through, and I noticed that the parents didn't intervene. Experience had taught them that constant reprimands had little effect, so they prudently held back.

Since then I've seen many children with ADHD – and, as with autism, there's usually enough evidence on display to make a preliminary diagnosis before the parents open their mouths. As I've only half-jokingly described it before, if we're one minute into a consultation and I'm already suppressing an urge to give a child a slap, there's a pretty good chance I'm looking at ADHD.

The symptoms of that first patient of mine were classic:

- **Attention deficit:** inattention and great difficulty focusing on an activity for more than a few minutes.
- **Hyperactivity:** constant activity and fidgeting.
- **Impulsivity:** acting or reacting with little thought for consequences, including calling out in class, lashing out when annoyed, and getting frustrated when asked to take turns or share.

The parents had already figured out some things that seemed to help, including getting the boy outside and physically active – if only because three hours of running around left him worn out and thus a little calmer. Their boy could also focus for slightly longer periods on some activities that were of special interest to him, such as helping his father fix the lawnmower.

All the same, they were at their wits' end. The school had lost patience with their son's constant off-the-wall behaviour, and so had they. They didn't know what to do next. Nor, to be honest, did I.

I felt I had little to offer, so I went away and did a lot of reading about how doctors abroad were dealing with the rising number of children turning up with ADHD symptoms.

The answer I found was one that made some people uncomfortable then, and still does today: that for the large majority of children with ADHD, judicious use of low-dose stimulant drugs is highly effective. The most widely prescribed drug is methylphenidate (better known as Ritalin and half a dozen other trade names), and there are also dextroamphetamine and amphetamine, each of which have multiple brand names.

As ADHD drugs began to be prescribed in New Zealand in the 1980s, many parents – and society in general – reacted with unease to the idea of drugging children and 'putting them in a chemical straitjacket'. I suspect amphetamine's reputation as the recreational drug 'speed' has added to those concerns.

I have always been wary of overmedication. My mother was bipolar, or manic-depressive as it was called at the time, and apart from the difficulties she and the rest of our family faced during her severe depressive episodes, I realised later that she had also been a victim of overprescription of assorted antidepressant and antipsychotic drugs. It seemed that for every symptom she had there was another drug to take, and then another drug again for the side effects. I realised that reaching for the prescription pad to satisfy patient demand could sometimes do more harm than good.

But in the case of ADHD, although I remained cautious I became increasingly confident that reaching for a pill was justified. What helped me change my mind, aside from the dramatic improvements I was seeing in children who were prescribed Ritalin, was that the parents of an ADHD child would have other children who showed no sign of it – which suggested it had little to do with parenting or the home environment.

The first time I said to a mother, 'This behaviour is intrinsic to your child – it's not that you are an incompetent parent,' she burst into tears. I wondered what I had said wrong, but she said they were tears of relief. She said she'd been feeling awful because she thought it was her fault as a parent.

I have heard this many times over the years. I think it is important to tell parents that although we can teach them strategies to improve their parenting, it is not bad parenting that caused their child's behaviours.

There is usually a genetic component. If you look back through a family's history, you'll find there is a pattern – perhaps a father or grandfather who was intelligent and capable but was never able to cope with the sitting-down-in-the-office parts of his job.

One question I sometimes ask is, 'How old was your son when he first climbed onto the garage roof?' Often the reply comes back quickly and without thought – 'About 10 months'. They don't even think the question is weird, because climbing onto the garage roof is what all kids with ADHD do sooner or later.

One woman who had recently remarried brought her 10-year-old stepson to see me, because she thought his behaviour was appalling. I agreed. His seemed a clearcut example of

ADHD. But the boy's father didn't see a problem. 'Oh,' he said, 'that's just how I was when I was young.' Which would be fine – except that as a teenager and young man the father's behaviour had been so reckless and impulsive he'd spent time in prison, and it was only in his forties that he'd finally settled down.

I convinced the father that I could help them find a dose that wouldn't completely dampen his son's enthusiasms and energy and zest for life, but *would* allow him to concentrate for periods long enough that he could start achieving some of his goals, in and out of school. We agreed on a six-week trial, starting during the holidays, which gave us time to get the dosage right before school started.

Within a few days of the new term the boy came home with certificates for good behaviour, and the teacher pulled the mother aside one day to say 'I don't know what you've done, but you've got a different child here!'

That six-week trial is something I do with the majority of my ADHD patients, and nine times out of 10 parents are highly positive about the change, though we may need to fine-tune the dosage. Their child will be earning praise at school and making friends more easily, while at home there'll be a lot less bouncing off the walls.

WHAT CAUSES ADHD?

There is one group in our society who, almost without exception, display the characteristics of ADHD. They are impulsive, inattentive and hyperactive. They want everything *now,* and won't take no for an answer. They have trouble considering the needs of anyone but themselves, and they're constantly busy.

This group are called two-year-olds, and delightful as they might be, it's a bit of a relief when they grow out of it all. You could say that ADHD is normal behaviour with abnormal timing, because when these toddlerish traits don't diminish with age, they become a problem worthy of a label and treatment.

Quite often, a child with ADHD will say they would like to be good, and hold back from shouting out in class, or roaming from their seat, 'but I can't help it'. This is very different to a child with straightforward bad behaviours. Some of the more enlightened teachers who've encountered a number of ADHD kids will refer to them as 'loveable rogues'.

About 3 to 5 per cent of New Zealand school-age children are affected by ADHD. Diagnosis rates are about three times higher in boys than girls, though it's not clear why. Girls may in fact be underdiagnosed because they seem more likely to have the attention deficit *without* hyperactivity (ADD), meaning they're dreamy rather than destructive. An ADHD boy who's throwing pencils around the room will get noticed faster than the girl who's away with the fairies at the back of the classroom.

A child with ADHD has real difficulty separating out the competing stimuli arriving through their eyes and ears and other sensory organs, and focusing on one thing at a time. If a child with ADHD is at their desk and there's a plane flying past the window, or someone walking outside, they'll likely forget the drawing or writing or focused listening they're meant to be doing and become distracted.

An ADHD child's high energy and thrill-seeking behaviour means they make friends fast but then lose them just as quickly because peers get sick of their bossy or wild behaviour.

Hyperactivity can cause social isolation, too. When birthday party invitations are being handed out, the child who always tears around popping the balloons and throwing cake is usually at the bottom of the list. (There's a tendency to blame sugar for the crazy behaviour that breaks out at children's parties, but in fact there is no evidence that sugar causes hyperactivity: the 'sugar-rush' phenomenon is mostly caused by the excitement of the group social interactions.)

IS ADHD BEING DIAGNOSED TOO OFTEN?

There is a view, which I don't totally dismiss, that ADHD in younger children is partly a matter of perspective. Many children, boys in particular, aren't ready for school at the age of five. They should be climbing trees and jumping in puddles rather than trying to sit up straight behind a desk.

I remember Ann coming home from a music lesson where one of our children was learning Suzuki Method violin. She said when some of the three- and four-year-old boys in the class started sword-fighting with their bows' a mother turned to Ann and said of her son 'He's always like that. We think he has ADHD,' and Ann thought to herself, 'No, that's just a four-year-old boy!'

It's hard to know whether the underlying rate of ADHD is rising, or just the diagnosis. In recent decades there has been increasing intolerance for boisterous behaviour and a rise in desk-based rather than physical work, so we may be picking up something that was there all along.

Despite all these caveats, the modern diagnosis and treatment of ADHD has been a godsend for many. These days people like that boy's father, who had to bounce around in the prison system as a teenager before he found his feet, would instead be given a small dose of

Ritalin and that chemical assistance would have seen him achieving at school, staying within society's guardrails, and not driving his parents to despair.

Because of my caution around overmedication I never made a formal ADHD diagnosis and prescribed a drug without first collecting information from three different places: I'd ask for a report from a behavioural psychologist, a report from the classroom teacher, and I'd also talk to the child directly.

This is very important, because some of the symptoms of ADHD are awfully similar to the effects of abuse, neglect or emotional upset. If a child is absolutely fine in school but a disaster at home, or vice versa, it's important to consider whether there's been bullying at school, abuse at home, or something else that needs to be unearthed. The classroom teacher report was much more revealing than the formal school reports, which are so sanitised and politically correct that they are unable to tell you anything that might possibly reflect negatively on the child.

One thing that would tip me towards recommending Ritalin when the diagnosis was borderline was if a child had become isolated from their peers because of their demanding behaviour. It's miserable to go through childhood being shunned in the playground, or left off those birthday invitation lists.

WHY DOES RITALIN WORK?

One of the functions of a part of the brain called the 'reticular activating system' is to help you focus, by filtering out extraneous stimuli that aren't relevant to the task at hand. When a person takes methylphenidate it stimulates neurotransmitter (in this case dopamine plus noradrenaline) activity in the reticular formation and in the front part of the cerebral cortex, thus improving that person's ability to focus.

Cynics might say 'Well, hang on, if you put everyone on Ritalin, everyone will be able to focus better.' That's quite possibly true – it's one of the many cans of worms that pharmacologists are prising open as they invent new drugs that promise to improve concentration, memory, creativity or motivation in healthy individuals.

Right now, though, the ethics of ADHD in children seem pretty obvious to me: we should only be giving drugs to children if there's a genuine, accurately diagnosed problem, and if the drugs have been shown to be effective and with an acceptable level of side effects.

Methylphenidate is a very short-acting chemical: it needs to be taken in several doses a day or in a slow-release pill. Within a short time of stopping taking it, the system is free of its effects – so many children take a break from the pills in weekends and holidays, when focused activity isn't quite as important.

WHAT ELSE CAN I DO TO HELP MY CHILD WITH ADHD?

Once you have a formal diagnosis that includes evidence that ADHD behaviours have been around for at least six months, your child may be prescribed medication such as Ritalin. But there are other things you can do as well.

- **One instruction at a time.** If you say, 'I want you to go upstairs, brush your teeth and then go tidy up your bed and bring down your jersey,' an ADHD child will do the first thing then get distracted and wander off. That's not going to change, so you're the one who's going to have to adjust.
- **Good routines, regular bedtimes.** Life with any child is easier if everyone knows the boundaries and rules, but for kids with ADHD it's especially helpful to have certainty around getting up, mealtimes, leisure, homework and bedtime.
- **Find the right teacher.** It's vital that your child's teacher understands ADHD and is understanding about the at times obnoxious behaviour it can cause. If the teacher isn't sympathetic, consider changing teachers – or even schools.
- **Manage your hopes around school and careers.** Some children with ADHD are

high-achievers, but many face additional educational hurdles, especially dyslexia. Many parents want a career for their child that's built on academic achievement, but some ADHD kids would be happier learning a trade where they could be using their hands. By adjusting your expectations, you may reduce some of the extra stress associated with the learning difficulties.

- **One-on-one time.** When life with your child has become a daily battle, taking the time to sit down and help them with something they really enjoy might be the last thing you feel like doing, but it's important for them to see that they can get your time and attention even (especially) when they're not acting out.
- **Food.** Don't get too anxious about sugar, preservatives and food colouring. Don't bother about food supplements. In fact, don't worry about food at all. Apart from the usual advice about having a balanced diet with plenty of fresh vegetables and not too much junk food, there is no good research to show that diet makes a scrap of difference to ADHD, and I'd argue that putting the entire family on a crank diet is just one more traumatic experience that you don't really need.

CEREBRAL PALSY

'We feel lucky – it could have been so much worse'

Jarrod was born at 28 weeks' gestation weighing about 1100 grams. That's young and small, but in NICU we've seen much younger and much smaller. But what unfolded over the following years was a demonstration of how a cerebral palsy diagnosis can creep up on you.

At Jarrod's six-month check there were no signs of physical impairment, but at 12 months he was 'toe-walking' (standing on tiptoes rather than flat-footed). Many children toe-walk for a little while as they develop towards normal walking, but it can also be an early warning of 'spastic diplegia' – cerebral palsy in the lower limbs – so we took note and waited.

At 15 months Jarrod's mother Sandy got back in touch: something about Jarrod's movement didn't seem right. When she brought him in I saw he was now quite noticeably tippy-toed, and my heart sank a little when I saw that his legs were quite stiff and his reflexes exaggerated. These were clear markers of spastic diplegia, albeit mild. Jarrod was a happy child, but he was clearly frustrated by his inability to walk and sit up unsupported. Still, I told Sandy, with the right therapy this might not be too severe.

We referred Jarrod for physiotherapy and orthopaedic surgeons, and he was given Botox injections. Botulinum toxin – the same stuff used to paralyse the facial muscles of people who want to lose their wrinkles – reduces muscle tightness. The downside is that it also causes some muscle weakness.

For Jarrod it was highly effective, and within 10 days of the injections he took his first steps. It was still not clear, though, how he would fare in the longer term.

WHAT IS CEREBRAL PALSY?

It's a condition where muscle movement in some part of the body is impaired as a result of brain or nerve injury sustained during pregnancy, during birth or immediately afterwards. It preys on the minds of many parents who come through NICU, seeing it is the most common neurological problem to affect preterm babies, and because at its worst it can be devastating.

At its mildest, cerebral palsy may result in little more than a slightly unusual walking gait, but it can also cause writhing, spasticity, muscle stiffness or floppiness and, in the most extreme (and fortunately rare) cases, a total inability to walk, talk – or both. Severe forms of cerebral palsy can be associated with intellectual disability, but milder forms are often not.

Severe cases may be obvious at birth, but milder cases won't always reveal themselves until the child has reached an age where they should be developing a new skill but don't, because the part of the brain that controls those muscles is damaged.

With these later diagnoses, parents may think their doctor missed something, but there may not have been anything to see. A problem with the arms, say, may not be apparent until the baby is five or six months old, when they should be starting to shove objects into their mouth but aren't.

WHAT CAUSES IT?

From the 1860s on, it was widely believed that cerebral palsy was always caused by perinatal asphyxia – a lack of oxygen at or around birth, causing brain inflammation and damage. In other words, it was the consequence of a difficult or bungled birth.

It would be more than a century before researchers showed that perinatal asphyxia was the cause of only 10 per cent of cerebral palsy cases. For the remainder, inflammatory damage in the baby's brain was present long before labour, and the difficult birth was possibly a *result* of the brain damage rather than the cause. This makes sense when you consider that some disruption of a baby's oxygen supply is almost inevitable during the squeezing and wrenchings of birth, and that the neonatal brain is built to cope with that kind of stress and recover quickly.

Sigmund Freud, better known for his innovations in psychiatry, guessed right in 1890 when he wrote that 'the anomaly of the birth process, rather than being a causal etiological factor, may itself be the consequence of the real prenatal pathology'. This long-standing overstatement of the importance of perinatal asphyxia has caused undue worry in many parents of children who needed resuscitation immediately after birth. The reality is that most resuscitated babies will feed well, go to the ward within hours and be healthy and back home within days.

HOW IS CEREBRAL PALSY TREATED?

The severity of cerebral palsy varies dramatically and so do the treatment options. One operation that's frequently performed on children with spastic diplegia releases tight Achilles tendons to make walking easier. Recovery from this includes time in plaster casts, which can be tough on the child – and also on parents.

Jarrod, the boy with spastic diplegia, is fortunate in having a determined personality that helps him cope with his frequent physical therapy and surgeries, and he has made slow but steady gains. He is now nine years old, plays touch rugby at school and mostly keeps up with his peers. He's of above-average intelligence and is a normal, happy kid, which includes being stubborn and obstinate at times and refusing to do what his parents ask.

Sandy has said she and her husband feel lucky when they see how much more severe cerebral palsy can be, but I can see that even this 'mild' case of cerebral palsy has been a hard road.

GLOBAL DEVELOPMENTAL DELAY

'Is my child keeping up?'

When Sarah's parents brought her to see me they were very anxious. At six weeks of age there seemed to be something badly wrong with their baby's ability to interact with the world.

Sit right in front of her and she would gaze over your left shoulder as if you weren't there. Change the lighting, make strange noises to get her attention, make silly faces – nothing seemed to draw her attention. After checking Sarah myself, I told her parents that the best thing to do right away was precisely nothing – or at least not yet.

I had seen babies like this before, and while it was conceivable that her visual inattention was a marker of something serious called 'global developmental delay', I was predicting a rather less worrying possibility – that Sarah's optic nerve pathways were getting off to a slow start, so not much information from her eyes was reaching her brain. That would change in time, and Sarah should eventually catch up.

We tracked her progress regularly. Each time, Sarah's vision had improved, even though she still lagged behind her peers. After 12 months, though, I was finally able to reassure her parents that Sarah's sight was entirely normal. She'd had a temporary lag in one facet of her development, but she got there in the end.

Most parents are familiar with the 'centile' growth charts that show the range of height and weight for a baby of a given sex and age, and let you compare your baby's progress with the population norms. You could create similar plots for any development milestone. When it came to vision, Sarah was one of those children whose numbers hovered around the third centile, which is at the low end of the normal range.

WHAT IS GLOBAL DEVELOPMENTAL DELAY?

This is when a child consistently fails to reach milestones throughout their life across all four broad areas of development: social/cognitive, speech/language, fine motor skills and gross motor skills. There are endless possible causes, including genetic abnormalities, brain injury and metabolic disorders.

If a delay is only in one area – in speech, say, or in gross motor skills – this is called 'developmental delay', and we usually adopt a 'wait and see' approach. In most instances, the child will catch up.

Even where it affects only one area, it is wise to identify a developmental delay as early as possible, as there may be treatments and interventions that can help. In the case of a language delay, it may be that the child's hearing is imperfect because of glue ear, and once that is sorted they're able to bounce back to where they should be.

Diagnosis can be tricky, however, for precisely the reasons shown in the case of Sarah: when a problem is first identified it may not be obvious whether it's a temporary developmental delay in just one area, or a warning of global developmental delay which is more likely to be there for life.

I was confident in Sarah's case because I'd seen this specific lag in vision numerous times before. I had been far less sanguine, though, the very first time I saw it, decades earlier. On that occasion I'd spent a lot of time and public money on high-tech investigations, including nerve conduction studies, brain scans and ophthalmology referrals, with a final good-news outcome identical to Sarah's.

Since then, in cases like this I have sometimes arranged for a second opinion from another specialist, probably to reassure myself as much as the parents that I'm not missing something more serious.

HOW DO I KNOW IF MY CHILD HAS GLOBAL DEVELOPMENTAL DELAY?

As a parent, worrying is part of the job description, so if you think your child is developing slower than expected at any time in their first few years, talk to your Plunket nurse or GP. They'll have a good idea of what's normal and what's not, and if they have concerns they should refer you on to someone who can conduct some tests.

It's important, though, that progress is monitored over time, as we did with Sarah. A snapshot in time is never as revealing or useful as a 'longitudinal' look – seeing a child several times over weeks and months. This gives a far clearer picture, and in most cases what seems like delay turns out to be a normal variation.

WHEN SHOULD MY BABY BE WALKING?

Some children walk at nine months, others nearer two years, with an average of around 13 months. Certain children are bottom-shufflers and become so proficient at it that they don't bother walking until long after they're physically able to do so.

When I was first practising I used to worry about late walkers and organise investigations, fearing the worst. Over time I realised that although the investigations were reassuring, they were mostly unnecessary; and that watching and waiting was more useful. Although in a child with global developmental delay walking will be one of many skills that arrive late, the age at which a baby walks is not generally predictive of later development.

In cases of concern a paediatrician will assess reflexes, the shape of the muscles and the tightness or looseness of movements. They'll also ask broader questions such as: At what age did the parents and siblings walk? Are there any other developmental issues of concern?

WHAT ABOUT SPEECH?

Speech is another of those milestones that parents worry about, sometimes unnecessarily. Much more important than speech or words is a child's understanding.

If a child can follow simple commands and make their needs known by pointing, grunting, nodding or leading you to what they want, we say they have 'language' rather than speech, and you can be fairly certain that the words will come. Another reassuring sign is 'conversational babble' – the delightful chatter that has all the intonation but none of the actual words of real speech (and often seems to happen at 5am when the child is standing in their cot, nattering away to no one in particular).

I am more concerned when a child doesn't even seem bothered that they don't understand a parent. Frustration about lack of speech is a good sign. A lack of interest in speech may herald an autistic disorder and is more concerning.

FOETAL ALCOHOL SPECTRUM DISORDER

'Is this one glass of wine OK?'

As referrals went, this was unusual: the would-be mother was only a couple of months pregnant, and when she walked into my office she was pretty sure she didn't want to have the baby.

She'd been to a wedding not long before, knocking back substantial amounts of champagne over a boozy weekend. Only later did she realise she'd been five weeks pregnant at the time. Now she was terrified that her unborn child was going to suffer from foetal alcohol spectrum disorder (FASD). She had asked her obstetrician for a termination, but he thought this was an overreaction and had referred her on to me for a broader discussion of the risks and realities of FASD from a paediatric perspective.

She told me she and her partner had been hoping to get pregnant around this time, so in principle they *did* want a baby. But she was terrified she'd damaged her foetus, having just read an article in a women's magazine with a headline along the lines of 'How I Destroyed My Newborn Baby's Future!'

I told her that in most cases where there is an occasional slipup in drinking alcohol while pregnant, the baby would be fine. After some discussion, she eventually accepted my reassurances and decided to carry on with the pregnancy. We wouldn't really know if all was well, though, until her baby was born.

WHAT IS FASD?

When a pregnant woman has an alcoholic drink the foetus also gets a few sips via the placenta. The wide range of physical and mental disorders that alcohol can cause in the growing foetus are collectively known as foetal alcohol spectrum disorder. Alcohol can disrupt the developing neural system as early as 20 days after conception, and other effects are probably caused much later in gestation.

The most extreme version of FASD is foetal alcohol syndrome (FAS), whose effects include problems with vision and hearing as well as cognitive functions, including memory, attention span and ability to learn.

A person with FAS will have stunted growth and distinctive facial features, including a flat nasal bridge, prominent eyes, a very thin upper lip and an absent philtrum (the double ridge between the nose and the upper lip). Heart defects are not uncommon.

In milder cases of FASD, the physical features aren't as obvious and the intellectual and behavioural effects can also be quite subtle, but include learning disabilities, hyperactivity, mood swings and an inability to assess the likely long-term consequences of behaviour (recklessness, in other words).

WHY ARE WE HEARING SO MUCH ABOUT FASD THESE DAYS?

There are accounts from ancient Greek and Roman times of the connection between consuming alcohol in pregnancy and abnormal babies, but foetal alcohol syndrome was only formally identified in the late 1960s, shortly before I started my medical training.

In 1982, the year I graduated in paediatrics, alcohol was confirmed as a teratogen (something that causes foetal malformation), based on research on non-human primates. Even then, the condition still hadn't been formally described in New Zealand (though it's safe to assume it existed). Just a couple of years later, in 1984, I encountered my first case – an adopted child called Luke, who had been slightly premature.

I wasn't the first to suspect that Luke might have FAS: it was his adoptive mother, who knew that the birth mother had taken drugs and alcohol in pregnancy, and had done some research of her own. Once she pointed out the characteristics in Luke I could only agree with her diagnosis. He had all the classic characteristics of FAS – small size, distinctive facial features and characteristic behavioural and intellectual problems, including ADHD, for which I eventually prescribed Ritalin.

The fact that I nearly overlooked my first case of FAS indicates the general lack of awareness of the condition at that time; and research by my colleagues Alison Leversha and Rosemary Marks later showed that the condition was being underreported in New Zealand, in particular.

Our oversight was partly because the symptoms can be quite subtle. But mothers also tend to understate the extent to which they drank while pregnant, and a child with FASD may well come from a tough family environment so behavioural issues were sometimes misattributed to social rather than biological factors.

Later I would gain a deeper understanding of FASD from my work assessing Russian orphans adopted by New Zealanders. Alcohol abuse is a major problem in Russia, and some of these children were born to mothers who had gone through pregnancy consuming vast quantities of alcohol and precious little nutritious food. The severity of the symptoms in some of these children exceeded anything I have ever seen in New Zealand-born children.

Doctors worldwide have come to realise that FASD is a bigger issue than we thought. Some researchers say it's the world's leading preventable cause of intellectual and developmental delays. Here and abroad many cases that would have been overlooked or misdiagnosed in the past are now being identified as FASD. Fortunately campaigns to persuade pregnant women to avoid alcohol have raised public awareness.

SO – IS THE ODD GLASS OF WINE DURING PREGNANCY OK OR NOT?

I believe without a doubt that we should be advocating for zero alcohol in pregnancy. We simply don't know what is a safe amount for the baby, and it differs for each individual.

As recently as 2015, the Ministry of Health reported that almost 20 per cent of pregnant women in New Zealand are still drinking alcohol (that's the average; the figure is higher for Māori and lower for Pasifika and Asian women). Somehow we are not getting the message across that it is not cool for young women to drink vast amounts of alcohol, especially if they are or could become pregnant.

On the other hand, for most expectant mothers who have been drinking before they realise they are pregnant, a few glasses is unlikely to have caused serious damage, provided they stop immediately.

In cases such as these – and there are plenty – sensible reassurance is needed. No one wants eight months of wondering if they've caused deformities in their unborn child, and anxiety itself can be associated with negative outcomes in the baby.

The pregnant champagne-quaffing mother who had come to me in a panic eventually delivered a healthy, bonny boy who weighed a reassuring 4kg. I reviewed him several times in his first two years and he seemed absolutely fine. He did turn out to have ADHD, but it's impossible to say if that was connected to the drinking. What was obvious, however, was that his parents loved him and wouldn't have been without him.

IMMUNISATION AND A PARENT'S RIGHT TO CHOOSE

To jab or not to jab – there's really no question.

In 2002 a Seventh-day Adventist couple, Jan and Deborah Moorhead, were jailed for the manslaughter of their six-month-old baby Caleb. Caleb had been suffering from malnutrition, anaemia and vitamin B12 deficiency because of his mother's extreme vegan diet, but when Starship tried to give him the simple and lifesaving treatment of vitamin injections, his parents took him into hiding. There they treated him with herbal remedies in what they described as a 'test of faith'. During the trial, an expert witness said Caleb could have been saved as late as half an hour before his death, if only he'd been returned to hospital.

Deborah was six months pregnant when she was imprisoned, and understandably there was grave concern about her ability to make sensible choices for her next child. She was forced to have vitamin B12 injections while in prison, and when her healthy baby girl was born the child was taken into Child, Youth and Family (CYF) supervision, though she was directly looked after by a family member.

As a Starship paediatrician I was asked to supervise the baby girl's medical care, with particular attention to her vitamin B12 levels and nutrition. But then the foster parents – who were otherwise very caring and loving and easy to work with – indicated that they were against immunisation.

This was an entirely separate issue from the dietary obstinacy that led to Caleb's death. Legally a parent can refuse immunisation for their child, but as the person appointed by the state to monitor this baby's health, I couldn't countenance her missing out on the benefits of immunisation.

Long discussions ensued about both the pros and cons of immunisation, as well as the issues facing me as the paediatrician who had state responsibility for her care. We eventually agreed to immunise her and all was well.

Tussles between medical professionals and anti-vaccination parents seldom get as dramatic or heavy-handed as this; my lobbying of parents is usually focused on education and gentle encouragement. That doesn't mean that I'm not passionate about the issue. I get especially angry whenever I hear that a doctor or nurse has advised parents not to immunise their children – educated medical professionals should know better.

In New Zealand the proportion of children who have received all the appropriate immunisations for their given age is around 89 per cent, a lamentably low rate for a developed country. There are two broad reasons for this: one is inadequate access to healthcare, whether because of geographical or social isolation, a lack of education or the expense of getting to a doctor. The other is that a depressingly large number of well-educated, well-resourced people have either misinterpreted the literature or been sucked in by anti-immunisation disinformation and have actively chosen not to immunise their children.

I have some sympathy for people being initially wary of a process that does, after all, involve injecting healthy young babies with processed particles of viruses and bacteria, in a form that sometimes contains scary-sounding substances such as mercury. So I do my best to bring parents along with me by showing them the evidence that immunisation is both safe and effective, and explaining why skipping the jabs is a bad decision both for their individual baby and for the community at large.

WHAT DO YOU SAY TO PARENTS WHO DON'T WANT TO VACCINATE?

For me the simplest piece of evidence is that countries with the highest rates of immunisation, such as Japan, Israel, Sweden, Denmark, Germany and the Netherlands, have the best child health statistics – in terms of infectious diseases, accidents, cancers and cot deaths. What this says, regardless of the individual, is that for a population, immunisations are associated with better outcomes.

If statistics don't work, I can talk about the reality of the diseases you're exposing your child to if you refuse to immunise. I sometimes ask parents to look at videos of a terrified baby with whooping cough, so they can see how horrible and frightening it is for the child gasping for breath, let alone for the parents.

I've seen at first-hand many of the diseases that have been either eradicated or dramatically reduced by immunisation programmes – and they aren't pretty. I'm just old enough that as a child I had a friend with a gammy leg because of a bout of polio. There used to be regular epidemics in New Zealand of this crippling and incurable paralysing disease, but since the arrival of an oral vaccine in 1961 there have been just a handful of cases, and none at all since 2002 when we switched to a safer and more effective injectable vaccine.

As a paediatric registrar I performed innumerable lumbar punctures on children admitted with the extremely nasty meningitis that's caused by the bacteria *Haemophilus influenzae*. In our hospital we saw cases every single week. The disease is fatal in 5 per cent of cases, and a third of survivors suffer permanent brain or nerve damage. This carnage was almost completely arrested when the Hib vaccine arrived in the 1980s.

When I was in Saudi Arabia in 1985 I treated a child with tetanus, and am still haunted by the appalling and agonising muscle spasms and rigidity the child went through before they eventually died. That infection was a result of the regrettable Bedouin practice of applying camel dung to the newly cut umbilical cord – an unlikely risk in New Zealand. Yet the tetanus bacterium is endemic in New Zealand soil, and there have been more than 30 cases here in the past 20 years; in almost every case, the victim hadn't completed their full course of tetanus vaccinations. The disease is incurable, and one in 10 victims die of it.

Measles, which used to be seen as a miserable but inevitable childhood disease, has the potential to be extremely serious, even fatal. Common complications include pneumonia, ear infections and diarrhoea. About one in 100 sufferers ends up in hospital. One in 1000 will develop an acute brain inflammation that can cause permanent brain damage or death. And there can be a disastrous postscript: I have watched a child die of the rare, degenerative brain disease called subacute sclerosing pan-encephalitis, which shows up a couple of years after the initial measles infection in one in 100,000 cases.

Vaccination with two doses of the MMR vaccine is 99 per cent effective at preventing a child from ever getting measles.

I could go on, but you get the point: immunisation directly prevents a world of pain, suffering and death.

BUT ISN'T A HEALTHY LIFESTYLE JUST AS PROTECTIVE AS A JAB?

Some of the parents who opt out of immunisations do so for the best of motives. They want to bring their child up in a world free of the ills of modern life, so they feed them organically grown vegetables and avoid additives and colourings, or battery farmed eggs and farmed fish, or meat, gluten, wheat or dairy. Skipping relatively modern innovations such as immunisation can feel like part of the same picture.

What they're perhaps forgetting is that 100 years ago parents would have had six children on the understanding that only four of them might survive childhood, because they were liable to succumb to measles, whooping cough, polio or meningitis, or even tetanus or diphtheria. It is true that with improved hygiene, sanitation and healthy nutrition some of these diseases were on the wane anyway, but there is clear evidence that health is improved even further by immunisation against these infectious diseases.

Parents who opt out because they think these diseases aren't very common any more are relying on 'herd immunity': if everyone else has immunised their child, an infectious disease won't take hold in the community so the risk to your child is quite low. But this approach is not only selfish, it's risky: if enough people opt out, herd immunity drops to the point where outbreaks occur. This is precisely what happened with measles, mumps and rubella after misguided fears of the MMR vaccine took hold in New Zealand in the late 1990s.

WHAT ABOUT GIVING JUST THE MOST IMPORTANT VACCINATIONS?

Some parents refuse point-blank to immunise their children, and our conversation ends there. But sometimes a parent will suggest some sort of middle ground, by asking if they might perhaps give their child only the 'most important' shots, or give the MMR triple vaccine as separate shots, in the belief that this might be less taxing on a child's immune system.

To the first request I can only say that all the immunisations we give have potential benefits, so it's impossible to say which is most important. Take the lot!

To the second I point out that scientists have found no immunological benefit whatsoever in splitting the MMR jab into three injections. Plus it means your child is getting punctured by three times as many needles. And you'll have to pay through the nose to do it privately, seeing as the government isn't willing to fund this pointless alternative to the freely supplied MMR.

BUT IMMUNISATION SOMETIMES FAILS, SO WHY BOTHER?

With any vaccination, a small proportion of those receiving it won't develop adequate immunity against the disease. That's definitely not an argument for skipping jabs. For a start, it's statistically unlikely that your child will be one of those unlucky ones; and if they are, the herd immunity that comes from the universal immunisation around them will still help protect them.

We owe a collective social duty not just to these unprotected children but also to the small number of children who have suppressed immune systems, perhaps because they are undergoing cancer therapy or have an immunodeficiency disorder. Those children are put at risk every time an electively unimmunised child walks into a classroom carrying an infectious disease. Some countries – though not New Zealand – recognise the risk an unimmunised child presents to a vulnerable classmate in preschool or school and will accept only children who have proof of immunisation.

Adults who were born before the era of MMR jabs and who didn't gain immunity by catching these diseases while young are still liable to get them in adulthood. This carries other risks. Recent media coverage of a couple of All Blacks who'd contracted mumps discussed the games they were missing because of their illness, but didn't mention that the men were at risk of reduced fertility or infertility because mumps can cause testicular inflammation if contracted in adulthood.

***

When I was three years old I had whooping cough. The endless coughing and feverish nightmares were bad enough, but to top it all off I was taken for a ride in an unpressurised Tiger Moth biplane at Taieri airport, buzzing around at an altitude of 5000 metres for half an hour, because of the then-fashionable theory that the lower air pressure at high altitude would help treat the cough.

That terrifying flight is one of my earliest memories. I've no idea if it helped the cough, but I do know that after the whooping cough vaccine began to be widely distributed in the 1960s, aeroplane-based therapy quickly fell out of favour. Quite simply, vaccination works – and the more people who do it the safer the entire community will be.

Sadly, I suspect that the misguided campaigners of the anti-vaccination movement will always be with us, just as there will always be a hard core of conspiracy theorists who doubt the reality of the moon landing (and it doesn't help that the most powerful nation in the world is currently led by a conspiracy theorist who seems unable to sort fact from noxious fiction).

It does little good for the medical community to harangue, and perhaps alienate, the parents who have swallowed those myths. All we can do is calmly and patiently present the scientific evidence and, whenever necessary, debunk the inaccurate claims of the 'anti-vax' zealots. It's a great pity that we need to waste time and breath countering their claims, but the health of our children depends on it.

CHAPTER 6

DIAGNOSIS

Diagnosis is at the heart of any doctor's practice, and no matter how sophisticated the tools and technology used, it will always remain an art as well as a science.

It was 1975. I was a freshly qualified doctor living in London and squeezing in trips around Europe and North Africa whenever I could find a gap in my hospital roster. This time the destination was Crete, where I'd flown with two New Zealand friends whom I had met on my travels, Lyndy Stout and Ginette McDonald (who later found fame as 'Lynn of Tawa').

After a couple of days in Heraklion we were keen to escape the hordes of German tourists. We took a bus, then hitched a ride with a passing farmer, and ended up in a remote village on the northern coast. We'd just checked into a pensione and were heading off for a swim when there was a commotion: a five-year-old girl had slipped on the rocks and badly cut her finger. I offered to help, and once the wound was stitched her family invited us to join them for lunch.

The set-up was almost too classical to be true: an extended family of 20 or so at an outdoor table beneath the vines in the garden of a rustic taverna. The girl's family were Athenians visiting their holiday home on Crete for the long weekend in celebration of some religious festival, and though we spoke no Greek and they no English, we had enough Italian and French between us to get by. What communication gaps remained were soon bridged with copious quantities of retsina, 'domestica' red wine and ouzo.

By late afternoon we were all firm friends – and thoroughly drunk – and the three of us had cancelled our pensione and accepted an invitation to spend the night at their holiday home a little further along the coast. We poured ourselves into a convoy of cars and took a hair-raising ride along the cliffs. I remember admiring the extraordinary colours in the sky as the sun began to set, and calmly wondering if this might be how my life would end: the driver was at least as drunk as me.

It was dusk when we arrived at their village, and café tables filled with patrons were spilling out into the main street. As we wended through this obstacle course, my driver nudged one of the tables, overturning chairs and knocking two men to the ground. I realised that one of the men, who was writhing on his back and clutching his arm, had a dislocated shoulder: I recognised the characteristically distorted bone and muscle beneath his skin. I knew how much pain he was in, as I'd had an identical injury through coming off my motorcycle while riding in Germany a year earlier. (I still recall how I screamed and swore at the staff at Überlingen Hospital as they popped the dislodged bone back into its socket.)

For the second time that day my medical training came in handy. As a surprisingly friendly crowd gathered round, I looped a towel below the man's armpit on the injured side and handed the ends back to Ginette so she could provide counter-traction. I then took off my shoes, lay down top-to-tail beside the man and put my foot into his armpit. I took his forearm with two hands and while Ginette hauled one way, I hauled the other until, with a heart-stopping thud, the shoulder snapped back into place. The man, who was about my age, gave a roar of pain as the joint graunched, but once it was back in place the relief was instant – though we still sent him to the local hospital to get treatment for the painful swelling that would inevitably follow.

The crowd cheered, I was handed another drink, and we were bustled off to the local hall, where the long weekend's festivities were in full swing. Later that night I and the doctor who'd treated the patient at hospital were prodded to the centre of a large circle of people and I was taught a *Zorba the Greek* -style dance, after which there was more applause and cheering. And drinking. (Looking back now, I wince at our recklessness, and am very grateful that this egregious drink-driving didn't result in something much more serious.)

The next morning I woke in a room with white walls and blue windowsills and shutters, and an alluring view of the sparkling sea. After a quick swim with one of my many new friends, Gianni, I was heading to the kitchen for breakfast when I saw that a queue had formed at the door.

After my public orthopaedic demonstration in the main street, half a dozen villagers figured I might be able to help them with their ailments, too. There was a sore throat, a person suffering from anxiety, a case of eczema, another of arthritis and a few others I can't remember. Patient Zero was there too, seeking treatment for the ribs that were broken at the same time as his shoulder was dislocated.

I was barely a year out of medical school and had no medical equipment with me, let alone a licence to practise or prescribe, but helping these people out on that day in Crete felt like the least I could do. So for the next hour, with some translation assistance from Gianni, that's what I did – and because of Greece's liberal pharmacy laws my unofficial patients were able to buy the antibiotics and pain relief I recommended, even without a prescription. In its own way that sunny, hungover morning in Crete was one of the most rewarding diagnostic sessions I've ever done.

Equally satisfying was when my hosts told me there were ruins a five-minute walk along the dusty road from the village. I discovered that this was Gournia, the ruins of an ancient and perfectly preserved Minoan town that I had written a Greek history paper on at Otago University years before. As I walked among the ruins I reflected on how it was as if fate had directed me there.

***

Diagnosis is at the heart of any doctor's practice, and no matter how sophisticated the tools and technology used, it will always remain an art as well as a science.

To make a diagnosis you need knowledge of the pathologies that might explain the symptoms, and an ability to think laterally and ask the extra questions that will fill in the gaps. But first you have to hear what the patient – or, in the case of many paediatric consultations, the parent – is trying to tell you.

That means being polite and kind and empathetic and, most of all, being a good listener – sitting down and hearing their story without interrupting. Some of what you hear won't be useful, but some will. A patient with recurrent chest infections might mention they broke their leg 30 years ago, which is hardly likely to be relevant, but as you sift through their history you might learn there was an aunt with tuberculosis living in the house when they were a child, say, and that might be *very* relevant. As a diagnostician it's your job to recognise which small pieces of evidence are the important ones.

As a paediatric registrar in Oxford I was about to discharge a girl we'd been treating for a nasty chest infection. As her father picked her up he asked why she had a squint. I said we'd assumed she'd had a lazy eye from birth, seeing it had been like that when she was admitted and her mother hadn't said anything.

'No,' said the father. 'That is new.'

In a slight panic I arranged an urgent scan of her brain, which showed three cerebral abscesses – life-threatening, pus-filled infections. She was transferred to neurosurgery and, after an operation and antibiotics, made a complete recovery. We were left wondering what might have happened if the father hadn't volunteered that crucial piece of information and she'd been sent home with just a bottle of antibiotics for the chest infection.

In diagnosis, a good rule of thumb is that the common things occur most commonly. In other words, once you've collected some symptoms, your list of possible causes should start with the boring bread-and-butter options before moving on to the rarer and more fascinating ones.

New graduates – and I was no exception – are tempted to jump to exotic and unlikely conclusions, but the tedious reality is that if someone has stomach pain and diarrhoea they probably have food poisoning or infectious gastroenteritis rather than a rare pancreatic tumour. A patient with a cough and fast breathing is more likely to have a simple chest infection than cystic fibrosis.

All the same, over a long career you'll also see some unusual and surprising cases, and they're not always easy to spot.

Tom, a 12-year-old, was brought into my Auckland clinic by his mother because he'd been getting nauseous most mornings, and sometimes at other times of day too. I gave him a general examination and saw nothing too out of the ordinary. Given that he'd also vomited a couple of times my first guess was that the nausea might be gastroenteritis caused by the parasite giardia, which can lurk in the gut for months if not treated. I arranged for a stool test and wrote a prescription for an antiprotozoal antibiotic. If the drug worked, that in itself would be near-confirmation of the giardia diagnosis.

We were almost done, but I got the feeling Tom's mother wasn't convinced. So, partly to reassure her, I decided to do a few more tests – including the standard neurological exam, which incorporates a test for coordination. I held out my hand and asked Tom to touch the tip of my finger, then the tip of his own nose. I got him to do this several times in a row with each hand.

I noticed that Tom's right hand was quite wobbly, and asked if he was left-handed. He wasn't, and that was strange because coordination is usually aligned with handedness. I still wasn't too anxious, but I now had to consider whether there might be something neurological going on. Early-morning headaches are a classic feature of increased intracranial pressure from a brain tumour, and though I'd never heard of a tumour causing early-morning nausea, perhaps there was a connection.

I said, 'Let's do a quick MRI scan just to rule a few things out.'

That was a week before Christmas. The scan was a few days later, and the radiologist phoned me on 23 December to say the scan showed a tumour right in the centre of the brain, involving the third ventricle. I phoned paediatric neurosurgeon Andrew Law and asked for some advice so I'd be able to talk to the parents more knowledgeably. He said the tumour could be benign or it could be malignant; we wouldn't know until after it had been removed. He kindly offered to see Tom the following day.

I rang Tom's parents at home: 'I want to come and talk to you about the scan results. Can you both be there?'

I was ushered into the lounge, where I described the scan and said the neurosurgeon would see them in the morning. We hugged, a few tears were shed and I left feeling bad.

After that, things moved fast: Tom was admitted on Boxing Day and the surgery went well – the tumour was in a difficult place, but it was benign. A couple of weeks later he was back home. For years afterwards I would phone early in the New Year to see how Tom was doing, and I'm pleased to report he's a fine young man who's completing a business degree.

The lesson for me was that you can never be too thorough. I still sweat a little, wondering how things might have played out if I hadn't felt that twinge of doubt from Tom's mother; if I hadn't pursued the less likely possibility of a neurological problem; if I hadn't spotted the wobbling hand and ordered the MRI.

***

Though listening is vital, visual observation is just as important, especially when assessing a baby. Just by looking you can see whether a baby has a good colour, indicating healthy blood circulation and oxygenation; whether the baby has good muscle tone or is floppy; whether they are alert and looking about; whether they are stretching and yawning or are too tuckered out to do even that; whether their breathing is fast or laboured; whether their head looks too big or too small; whether they know how to calm themselves or are flailing their limbs aimlessly. Before I've laid a finger on the child, I've already gathered much of the information I need.

While making these quiet observations, I can also be talking to the parents, learning a little more about the family environment and what the parents themselves have noticed about their baby.

Some genetic and developmental disorders have such clear visual markers that a preliminary diagnosis can be made in seconds.

A couple brought their two-year-old son to see me because he had been suffering from diarrhoea, but before they started describing the symptoms I was fearing something much worse than a dodgy tummy. For such a young child he had an extremely mature face, almost like an adult's, and his skin had a swarthy Mediterranean look, even though his parents were Pākehā.

These were textbook symptoms of a class of metabolic disorders called mucopolysaccharidoses, which I recalled from my time at medical school. I arranged for a screening for the disorder and the results came back positive. The boy had a condition that invariably led to severe mental retardation and death at a young age – not easy news to break to the parents. The condition was one that could occur again, so the parents received genetic counselling; they later went on to have another, healthy child.

Even quite subtle aspects of a child's appearance can provide a lot of useful information. In a less politically correct time, obstetric and paediatric staff would sometimes use the shorthand of 'FLK' in a child's medical notes, meaning 'funny-looking kid'. Although it now seems unkind and offhand, at the time this wasn't meant as mockery or insult: rather, it captured the general impression, without getting too specific, that there was something about this child that merited a closer look. Now that we're more aware of the impact of careless words, we talk about 'dysmorphic' characteristics, but the ability to look at a child and think 'something's not quite right here' remains a powerful diagnostic tool.

Ella's mother brought her to see me because she was growing rather slowly, which her mother put down to her not eating well. The first things

I noticed about this little girl, though, were her cute little turned-up nose and pixieish face. She was in fact perfectly well nourished: her size, along with her distinctive facial characteristics, were symptoms of the genetic disorder Williams syndrome, where about 25 genes are missing from a specific chromosome, causing a constellation of developmental issues. Symptoms of Williams syndrome include some intellectual disability, though that's not always noticed until school age; children with the syndrome are often unusually sociable with a cheerful personality and excellent verbal skills.

Genetic tests confirmed my suspicion. Ella and her parents took it all in their stride: the diagnosis meant they knew what to expect in the coming years, and it was also helpful for getting extra learning support. Ella's parents know she has limited academic potential, but she's a thriving and happy girl.

For many people the most familiar dysmorphic features are those that indicate Down syndrome. Seen individually they can mean little or nothing, but together they add up to something: the gently slanted eyes, the small, flat nose with a missing nasal bridge, the fold of loose skin at the back of the neck, the widely spaced nipples.

For all my experience in this area though, first impressions can still be wrong. Once, after checking on a newborn baby I had an inkling she might have Down syndrome but it wasn't clearcut. I wrote about it in the child's notes, intending to take a closer look the next morning. But that evening the father picked up her notes and spotted that I'd written 'trisomy 21?'

I was called back to the ward to explain the note to the parents, and had to admit that I wasn't sure whether their girl had Down syndrome or not. I said certain clues in her face had raised my suspicions but, until it became more than a hunch, I hadn't wanted to worry them unnecessarily.

By the next morning the baby was looking more normal to me, and with each day I grew more confident that she didn't have Down syndrome. After five days I was certain, but the parents were still anxious so we sent a gene test off anyway. It came back negative and the baby went home. Just before they left, the mother told me the false alarm had been very unsettling: 'I don't know whether I'll ever be able to look at my baby the same way.'

Those words really stuck with me, because they captured a common dilemma: if you're not yet sure about a diagnosis, do you really need to tell the parents about every possibility – dire or otherwise – that's bouncing around in your head?

Forty years ago, when paternalism from doctors was not only accepted but expected, the typical approach was to say nothing at all if you suspected a baby had Down syndrome and to quietly send off for a gene test, which back then took a couple of weeks. By the time the test came back, most parents would have totally bonded with their child, would love them to bits and wouldn't reject them, no matter what the result.

The idea here, as one of my professors put it during my training, was that you don't want to ruin those precious first few days or weeks – so if there is an abnormality, why not let that information emerge at its own pace?

Today the patient's (or the parents') right to know is absolute. By telling them everything we know as soon as we know it we are, arguably, slightly increasing the risk of rejection, but I don't think that's a good enough reason to withhold information.

***

Long ago, an obstetrics colleague said to me: 'If you're around for long enough, you'll get complaints. It's not a matter of how good or bad you are. It's a matter of how much work you do.'

Some complaints I've received, however, have forced me to reflect on my diagnostic methods and bedside manner. One related to a check-up of a seven-year-old boy. I can't even remember why his mother brought him to see me at my paediatric clinic – perhaps a chesty cough or a sore tummy. In any case I was giving him all the usual checks: take his blood pressure, listen to his chest, palpate his tummy, check reflexes, a quick look in his eyes and ears and a check of his genitalia.

I was pulling his shorts down while saying something bland like 'Let's have a quick look here' when the mother asked, 'Why are you doing that?'

I said, 'It's just part of the routine examination.'

'Well he doesn't like it,' she replied.

To my eyes the boy couldn't have cared less that a doctor had briefly tugged down his pants while his mother sat nearby, but I said nothing, finished the exam and that was that.

Except a few weeks later I was notified by the Medical Practitioners Disciplinary Tribunal that a formal complaint had been made against me.

In my response I pointed out that undescended testes is a not uncommon condition, and is one of the standard things I rule out the first time I examine a young boy. The consequences of *not* spotting it can be dire, including infertility and an increased risk of testicular cancer; and if he had it and I didn't spot it, I would rightly be exposed to accusations of negligence.

The conversation went back and forward, with the mother saying I should have given more warning of what I was about to do and me responding that with boys that age it was better to be matter of fact than to turn it into a big embarrassing conversation.

In the end my insurance company, which would have had to deal with any financial fallout if the argument continued, asked me to write a polite letter of apology to make the problem go away. I did as I was asked, but not without a certain amount of steam coming out my ears. My letter said, in paraphrase, 'Sorry I upset you. Here's why I did it. I promise not to do it that way again.' I still considered I had done nothing wrong, and I didn't really change my methods – but I am now more careful about checking with a parent first.

I had to defend myself in another case when a mother sent a letter complaining that I'd gone off-topic during her daughter's consultation. The girl, who was about nine, had come in with a fairly minor respiratory problem, but as we chatted away I'd changed the subject somewhat. The girl was seriously overweight, and I started showing her the graphs of where she should be for her height and age, and quizzing her a little on what she knew about good food and bad food. I suggested that at her age it would be a great time to start thinking about the types of food and drink she was consuming.

The girl seemed interested and receptive. But I then got the letter from her mother, saying she was extremely upset that I had ambushed her and her daughter with a lecture about obesity.

I am always pretty careful when talking about weight with children, especially with girls, and especially once they've reached the age of 12 or 13. That's the age at which, for reasons that aren't well understood, girls become liable to develop anorexia nervosa, bulimia and other eating disorders; and insensitive comments, however well-meant, can trigger pathological eating habits.

Yet obesity is the largest health crisis facing children today all around the world. If we don't do something our hospital wards will be full of people with diabetes, heart disease and other obesity-related illnesses. Clearly the obesity epidemic must be tackled at multiple levels. I suspect the best long-term solutions will arise from bold political action – urban design and transport planning that puts exercise back into our everyday lives; regulations that rid school tuckshops of junk food and move dairies further away from the school gate; bans on junk-food advertising; and greater pressure on food manufacturers and distributors to change their recipes and price structures so it's healthy food that's cheap and easy, not sugary drinks and fat-laden convenience foods.

While high-level organisational and political lobbying are vital, doctors in the community are uniquely positioned to lobby directly the people who are most at risk.

When a doctor is talking to a child between the age of eight and 10, they have a rare opportunity to deliver a bit of positive propaganda to an entire family. It's an age where the child is still young enough to have some respect for the authority of an adult, but old enough to have the confidence to pressure their parents. A nine-year-old will say 'Look, the doctor said...' and suggest that the family skips the McDonald's or the home-fried foods in favour of something healthier.

I did send a reply to this mother as well, saying 'sorry you were offended' and explaining my reasons. I realise that when you couch an apology in that way it's barely an apology, but in truth I was reluctant to grovel too much simply because I'd talked to a nine-year-old about a few small changes she could make to improve, perhaps even save, her life. That is basic health advocacy.

***

When I was about eight some townie friends of my parents came to the farm for lunch, bringing their daughter Susan and, much more interestingly, Susan's new toy, a doll called Flubber. The doll's selling point was that he was indestructible. Made of sponge rubber and metal, he could be bent and folded and withstand any insult. I was fascinated, and persuaded Susan that we should take Flubber to the woodshed and put his indestructibility to the test with an axe.

The first swing bounced off the foam rubber, but at the second blow the blade snapped through the wire internal frame and chopped Flubber completely in half. Shocked, we guiltily hid Flubber's remains under the back seat of her parents' car, and lied through our teeth when it was time for them to leave and Flubber couldn't be found.

Though my ethical standards have improved since then, I like to think that the day I investigated Flubber's innards represents a milestone in my lifelong curiosity about how the body works, and a determination to figure out what makes things tick.

It was this kind of curiosity that drove me to plough through a rather dry book called *Mechanics of the Motor Vehicle* when I was 13. I wasn't especially good at maths or science, but I really wanted to know how cars worked, so I read and reread it until I understood the principles of getting petrol to ignite, produce energy, push a piston up and down to produce rotation, then using the camshaft to convert the axis of rotation and make the wheels spin.

The same curiosity would later inspire bursts of enthusiasm where I'd read for hours until I knew, say, the rudiments of the stars and planets, or the names of all the New Zealand native trees and shrubs. In my mid teens, my fixations broadened to include poetry. I suspect that my father, as well as his farmworkers, were slightly baffled that I spent my smoko breaks during haymaking reading Gerard Manley Hopkins, Dylan Thomas and Robert Frost.

I believe that the art of medical diagnosis is built on that kind of curiosity. When training young practitioners now, I tell them diagnosis must always include not only the question 'what' but also the question 'why'. A 'why' will guide you towards asking the right questions and developing a more complete understanding of a condition. What's more, when you ask 'why' you create an opportunity to prevent something happening again.

It was asking 'why' that led to Jane Harding's identification of the dangers of chest physiotherapy on premature babies. And it was asking 'why' that led a pair of Auckland researchers to solve the mystery of an epidemic of stillbirths among Pasifika babies.

In the mid-1980s, Auckland hospitals started seeing extraordinarily high rates of stillbirth among babies born to mothers who were immigrants from the Pacific Islands. Many were full-term babies of a good size who had died or were left with major permanent brain damage, due to inexplicable brain bleeds. I saw a number of these babies immediately after birth, and their injuries were shocking.

Researchers Tania Gunn and David Becroft analysed 47 such cases and concluded that the deaths were caused by a traditional pregnancy massage, practised in Tonga and Samoa especially, that involved trampling over the pregnant mother's belly.

Gunn and Becroft's findings sparked a vigorous education programme within Pasifika communities both in New Zealand and back in the mothers' home countries. The massage technique swiftly fell out of favour and, in Auckland at least, the prevalence of that kind of injury swiftly fell to zero.

***

I have seen from both sides how infuriating and upsetting a poor diagnosis can be.

In 1994 I was living in Auckland when my father rang from Otago to say he'd been unwell. He'd had slurred speech and facial weakness and a weak arm, and though he'd since recovered he said his GP had told him he must have suffered a small stroke.

I was very surprised that he would have had a stroke when he'd not had high blood pressure or other common risk factors such as diabetes or obesity. Over the phone I switched into doctor mode and asked him if there had been anything else going on with his health recently.

'Well,' he said, 'I haven't been able to get warm all summer, and I've had some back pain.'

Dad was a lifelong heavy smoker. This information indicated to me that rather than a stroke, something much more sinister might be going on, such as a cancer with cerebral and spinal secondary tumours. I insisted he see a neurologist, and after further investigation it turned out the worst was true. Dad died nine weeks later.

Although the misdiagnosis didn't make a long-term difference to the outcome, I was furious that his GP hadn't had the curiosity to ask why a previously healthy 71-year-old man, without the right risk factors for stroke, should have had one at all.

The question he'd failed to ask was, 'Why?'

CHAPTER 7

FROM RUSSIA WITH LOVE

Conducting long-distance paediatric assessments of Russian orphans was a tiny yet surprisingly enjoyable sideline to my regular work.

The video is just a few minutes long, and although it's in colour it's dimly lit and the image isn't very sharp. It shows a young girl, maybe two years old, holding a toy. Heartbreakingly, she is a little unsure what to do with it. In another short clip a female caregiver is talking to her, but she's not getting much response from the little girl. The child looks healthy enough, and from what I can see of the background the orphanage seems clean and warm. The girl's head looks a little smaller than average for her age, but that isn't unusual – and may not be as ominous as it seems.

I watch the video in my office, then a couple more times that evening, looking carefully for all the little visual clues: Does the little girl appear socially interactive? Is she using all her limbs? How do her fine motor skills seem? How's her posture? Her gait? Are there signs of genetic abnormalities, or any of a number of developmental syndromes? Is she acting the way you'd expect for a child of her stated age? I weigh up what I'm seeing and compare it against the brief notes, translated from Russian, that I've also been given.

Tomorrow an anxious pair of would-be parents will want to hear my opinion, and then they'll have only a few days to make their decision because they've already booked their flights. On the sparse evidence in front of us, should they adopt this child from a Russian orphanage and bring her to New Zealand for a new life, or leave her to her fate?

***

After the USSR collapsed in 1991, the world became aware of the plight of an estimated 300,000 children living in orphanages in Russia. Over the next 20 years, Russian orphans were adopted by parents from all over the world before regulatory changes there made it nigh on impossible. Around 700 of those children were adopted by New Zealanders.

Conditions in Russian orphanages were nowhere near as bad as those in Romania where, after the collapse of the Ceaușescu regime in 1989, it was discovered that orphanage inmates were being routinely abused, drugged and tied to their beds or starved to death. All the same, standards weren't great in Russia: inadequate staffing meant children under three in particular were receiving far less one-on-one attention than they needed.

Many were 'social orphans' – meaning they had ended up in state care not because their parents were dead but because they were too poor, substance-addicted or otherwise unable or unwilling to care for them. Foetal alcohol spectrum disorder (FASD) was distressingly common, including extreme cases. Sometimes children with a problem that in New Zealand would be considered minor had been abandoned by Russian parents who couldn't afford treatment or couldn't face raising a 'disabled' child.

The process of bringing a Russian orphan to New Zealand was complex and difficult; it might involve multiple trips to Russia, and could cost $50,000 or more. Yet plenty of would-be parents were willing to give it a go, not least because there were virtually no local New Zealand children available for adoption. From the 1970s on, widespread availability of contraception and abortion, plus the sweeping social and political changes that removed the stigma of women having a child outside of marriage, meant local adoptions dried up. In 1971, 4000 New Zealand children were put up for adoption; by 2016 that figure had fallen to 128 children. That same year there were 745 children adopted from abroad.

I got involved with the Russian orphans because parents wanted a professional opinion about the health and prospects of the child they were considering adopting. From the mid-1990s, I saw six to 12 cases a year for a couple of decades. The parents – mostly from Auckland but some from as far afield as Gore or Dunedin – would come to my private practice with the medical records of a child and, more often than not, a short video, the practical value of which varied widely.

I was already familiar with assessing children who were destined for adoption, though under rather less exotic circumstances. From 1986 I was the visiting paediatrician to Bethany Home in Grey Lynn in central Auckland. Run by the Salvation Army, this was a place where young women, most of them teenagers, came to live in the latter stages of their pregnancy and for a few weeks after their child was born, usually with the expectation that the child would be adopted out (though a small number of mothers held on to their child). It was a wonderfully supportive and safe environment for these young women.

My role was to 'approve' the children as fit and healthy for adoption. As a rule these well-cared-for babies were just that – fit and healthy. If I found a minor medical issue I would make sure the adoptive parents were alerted and knew what follow-up might be needed.

Personally assessing a newborn New Zealand baby at a teen maternity home a few miles from my home was a very different proposition from what I was doing for the prospective parents of the Russian orphans. Some of the videos they brought along were less than a minute long; others were 20 minutes. Sometimes the parents had already been to Russia and had made the video themselves, so they already had a good idea of what they were dealing with. In other cases they were as much in the dark as me, trying to make a preliminary decision about a child based on some blurry videos and a sheaf of papers.

The files were in some ways harder to interpret than the videos. As a matter of policy, some orphanages would release children for international adoption only if they had serious physical or developmental problems. As a result, medical staff would sometimes overstate a child's disabilities to smooth their passage to a better life abroad. I learnt how to read between the lines, knowing that the negative features had been embellished. Many children would be described as having suffered severe perinatal asphyxia, putting them at risk of cerebral palsy, but when I looked at other details such as birth weight and Apgar scores (a 10-point scale that grades the appearance and behaviour of a newborn to assess the need for resuscitation), it would be obvious that the asphyxia was a fiction. A child might be described as having major language delay caused by deafness from untreated glue ear when, in fact, the glue ear had been cured long ago with no lasting ill-effects.

On the other hand, some children were genuinely disabled or showing clear signs of FASD, so I couldn't simply dismiss out of hand the dire warnings in the notes. I had to be careful, too, about how I interpreted what I was seeing. One of the things I was looking at closely was head size: a small head can be an indicator of a range of different problems, including FASD. But a small head is also associated with a lack of nurture: if a baby or young child isn't receiving all the attention, cuddles and parental chatter they need, their brain – and thus their head – will grow more slowly than it should. This can be a temporary problem if the undernurtured child receives remedial doses of love and attention before they get too old. Sometimes, though, it wasn't easy – based on some deliberately misleading medical notes and a short, grainy video – to know which kind of small head I was looking at.

Parents were justifiably anxious about the prospects for a child. The international adoption process had been rather tainted by the Romanian orphanage scandal where, on top the appalling general neglect and ill-treatment of infants, many had been given blood transfusions to 'boost their strength' and the blood turned out to be infected with the HIV virus, with devastating consequences. Around 160 Romanian orphans came to New Zealand, though I was not involved in any of their assessments.

I was as accurate in my assessments of the Russian children as I could be: I would be honest if I thought there were serious developmental problems, and positive if I thought a problem was small enough to overcome.

I remember the video of an especially lively one-year-old boy with dark brown eyes and olive skin who had an engaging, enquiring personality that made him stand out. However he had a cleft lip and palate, which can be quite confronting and hard to look at if you're not used to it – the inside of the upper mouth and nose appear to be inside out. I was keen for him to be adopted to New Zealand where surgery would have been immediately available and would, in time, leave him looking completely normal and able to fulfil his potential. If he stayed in Russia he might never have the defect corrected, and he was already getting past the ideal age for surgery. Unfortunately, the prospective parents couldn't bring themselves to adopt him. I hope that someone else was able to do so.

If a child I'd assessed did make it to New Zealand I would meet them in person and perform a standard assessment of their development, as well as weighing and measuring them, checking their immunisation status and testing for HIV and hepatitis, as well as giardia, which was surprisingly common. The youngest child I assessed was nine months old; the oldest five or six years. Six months and 12 months later I would repeat the assessments, and I was almost always blown away at the progress I would see.

Sacha was pretty typical of the children I saw – a tousle-haired blond four-year-old with blue eyes, who had seemed physically healthy but rather withdrawn when I first saw him on video. I met him a couple of weeks after his arrival in Auckland when he came in with both of his new parents. He was very shy; he spent a lot of time on his mother's knee (itself a good sign of a developing attachment) and was reluctant to explore the toy box. His mother had learnt a little Russian to talk to him, but he was already picking up English at a rate that astounded me.

At this first meeting I had a feeling that some of his diffidence was based on fear of being taken away again. I had to remind myself that in the space of about three weeks he had been plucked from the orphanage, moved into a hotel room with two complete strangers while the parents waited for his official papers, flown across the world in an aeroplane (almost certainly his first flight ever), taken to a new home full of toys and pets and other luxuries, and had started preschool. He was no doubt wondering whether all this was to be a permanent arrangement or not.

At the follow-up meeting six months later he was fluent in English and you'd have been hard-pressed to tell that he wasn't an everyday New Zealand-born child. Most striking of all, though, was the change in one simple measurement: the size of his head.

The first few times I did the follow-up measurements on a Russian orphan I thought I must have mischarted the initial figure, but after it happened several times I realised that these children were simply making up for the ground they'd lost during their understimulated months or years in the orphanage. Time after time their head measurements – a rough proxy for the size of the brain inside – would leap up through the centile charts.

In general, the younger a child was adopted, the more likely they were to catch up neurologically and settle in emotionally. I also found that if the child had had a sibling in the orphanage they were more likely to adjust well subsequently. I presume this was because having an attachment to a sibling as opposed to a parent is still preferable to having no attachment figure at all.

Most parents I met worked to maintain a connection with their child's home country, including trips back to Russia. International adoption has its critics, but I firmly believe that if the choice is between living your formative years in an orphanage versus having a loving family environment in another country, the latter is what is best for the child.

Though my long-distance assessments proved mostly accurate, I always warned prospective parents of the risk of missing something when working from such superficial data, and of problems that might not show up until later. I also urged them to keep this risk in perspective. Whenever anyone embarks on a pregnancy they have to accept that their child may not be perfect, or may even turn out to have major problems, but we accept the lot that we are given. So it is when adopting.

On one occasion a little girl whom I'd assessed developed severe cerebral palsy. Her mother was very miserable about this, and more than a little angry at me. We had both understood that there was always the possibility of this happening, but that didn't stop me from feeling awful about it too.

New Zealand media have given us intermittent snapshots, both positive and negative, of the lives of some of those Russian orphans. In the early 1990s there were interviews with thrilled parents returning from their Eastern European odyssey, and every few years there would be a follow-up story about how the children they'd brought with them were settling in. A few of the adoptive parents were public figures, such as politician John Banks and his wife Amanda, who adopted three siblings from a St Petersburg orphanage in 1995.

Both here and abroad, however, there were some more-troubling stories. In 2010 a woman in Tennessee created international headlines when she put her seven-year-old adopted grandson on a one-way flight back to Russia, saying he was mentally unstable and had profound 'psychopathic' behavioural problems that had been lied about by the orphanage staff when she and her daughter had collected the boy a year earlier.

In 2014 a young Christchurch man appeared in court to face five charges after a 'mini crime spree' in Akaroa: two burglaries, two thefts from cars and driving without a licence. The judge noted that the young man had suffered significant emotional deprivation in his first two years in a Russian orphanage, which had left him with an attachment disorder that was virtually impossible to treat despite the best efforts of his adoptive parents and various therapists. At 20 he already had a lengthy criminal record, and he had once held the dubious honour of being Christchurch's most prolific youth car thief.

This kind of long-term dysfunction is an adoptive parent's worst nightmare, and an acknowledged risk: the very reason these orphans needed new homes was that they were, in general, undernurtured, and thus at risk of attachment disorder. Such extreme outcomes are rare, but in a 2013 article on international adoption, Child, Youth and Family was quoted as saying a 'handful' of overseas adoptees had ended up in its care, presumably because of behavioural problems that were too much for the adoptive parents.

I haven't stayed closely in touch with many of the families I helped, but among those whose progress I have followed, things have gone well – mostly.

One child, James, had a small head at the time of my first assessment, and I discussed the real risk that he had foetal alcohol syndrome. Once he'd reached New Zealand we confirmed that this was the case, but his new parents knuckled down to the job of doing their best for him. At primary school he was a handful and needed teacher aide assistance, and I later diagnosed him with ADHD and started him on Ritalin. He went through another tough patch in adolescence – running with a bad crowd and being socially immature – but once again his parents helped him through it. I recently spoke to his father, who said he's settling down, though he still definitely needs his Ritalin.

It's important to remember that you don't need to be a Russian orphan to go through a rough patch during adolescence. One family I hadn't heard from for more than a decade got in touch in a bit of a panic: their adoptive son, now 16, had met up with a friend and the two of them had polished off a bottle of vodka, ending up seriously intoxicated.

Was this, they worried, the past come to haunt them – bad behaviour linked to attachment disorder, or some echo of alcohol abuse in the birth family (it was vodka, after all!)? I had a chat with the boy and did a full adolescent health assessment including a HEADDSS questionnaire (health, education, activities, drugs, depression, sex, suicide). It was clear he was an ordinary, well-adjusted kid who'd made a dumb decision that was far more likely due to the fact that he was a high-spirited teenager than because he was an orphan. He and his mate had just been playing up – behaving in a way that was pretty familiar to me as a father of three teenage boys of my own.

Other reunions have been sweeter still: I was at a classical music concert in the city when a young man came up to me and introduced himself as one of those kids I'd met fresh off the plane from Russia. He was now an arts student with a passion for music, and was living a very happy and normal life.

***

Conducting long-distance paediatric assessments of Russian orphans was a tiny yet surprisingly enjoyable sideline to my regular work, and when the rules of international adoption started changing in Russia around 2006 I was sad to see the work end.

My work with the babies and mothers at Bethany Home dried up around the same time, not because New Zealand's teen pregnancy rate was falling but because mothers were choosing to hold on to their babies. I had mixed feelings about this because, without a lot of social and financial support, it's a tough road raising a child when you've barely finished your own childhood. The statistics show that unsupported teen mothers are much more likely than their peers to end up with no qualifications and to be dependent on benefits; and rates of depression, suicidal ideation and substance dependence are all higher.

It was a true pleasure to be able to help adoptive parents who were moving heaven and earth to get the child they so dearly wanted. In many cases there was a strong streak of altruism in their desire to give a child a better life, even though there was a risk they might be a handful.

It was also professionally satisfying. It was an interesting challenge to put together the most reliable and useful report you could, based on meagre and subtly unreliable data. Watching the videos and reading the reports was an exercise in perspective, reminding me how good the New Zealand health system is when you consider that, elsewhere, something as minor as a cleft-lip repair is unavailable to a child who desperately needs it.

I felt strangely privileged to have witnessed a sort of accidental neurological experiment: the brain growth and head size of virtually every one of these orphans accelerated dramatically once they'd been placed with their new, nurturing family – evidence that love and attention are the fundamental 'food' for brain growth.

It was an experience that would prove invaluable when, in the early 2000s, I became involved in a charity that would start to change the way child development was viewed by some of the most powerful institutions in the country.

CHAPTER 8

BRAINWAVE

In essence, if you can fill the first 1000 days of a child's life with cuddles, attention and kindness, you're setting them up for a happy, healthy and productive adulthood.

Imagine, for a moment, that someone tells you they've identified something in the environment so toxic that exposure to it triples your chances of getting cancer, and quadruples the odds of heart disease over the course of your life. Imagine being told that this thing is also linked to a twelvefold increase in the risk of suicide, a fivefold increase in depression, and has been implicated in some pretty nasty effects on brain development, the immune system, hormonal systems and other body systems besides. In sum, the doom merchant explains, exposure to this will knock an average of 20 years off your lifespan.

Surely you'd want to avoid exposure to this dread substance. And if you were a doctor, you'd possibly want to do something about keeping people safe from it.

Well, as Californian paediatrician Nadine Burke Harris explained brilliantly in a *Ted Talks* presentation that's been viewed online 3.5 million times, researchers have identified just such a danger in our environment, and it's 'not a pesticide or a packaging chemical'. It's childhood trauma.

Burke Harris was specifically talking about a piece of research conducted in the mid-1990s by the San Diego health insurance provider Kaiser Permanente and the US Centers for Disease Control. The study asked 17,500 people to fill in a simple questionnaire measuring their childhood exposure to 10 different types of adverse childhood experience (ACE), including physical, emotional or sexual abuse; neglect and exposure to family violence; parental addiction or mental illness; and loss of a parent through divorce, abandonment or incarceration. If you've experienced none, you score 0; if you've experienced all, you score 10.

The ACE scores were then statistically analysed alongside the detailed health history of each person. The results were extraordinary: a clear correlation between the ACE score and the extent of bad outcomes in almost every imaginable facet of health: cardiovascular disease, hepatitis, mental illness, immune problems, cognitive function, asthma, cancers, immune problems and more. For example, if you had an ACE score of 7 or more, you had triple the lifetime risk of lung cancer compared with someone with an ACE score of 0. And the effects of a high ACE score were shown to be quite independent of the fact that a difficult childhood means you're also more likely to be a smoker and a drinker and make other choices that hurt your health.

It's not exactly news that a tough childhood sets you up for a difficult adulthood, but the CDC–Kaiser ACE study was an important addition to a growing body of research that is revealing the lifelong impacts of childhood trauma, as well as the complex biological mechanisms that literally reshape the brains and bodies of children exposed to it.

Over the past 20 years, researchers around the world have been picking away at this problem from multiple angles. Evidence has been amassed from MRI scans of the brains of criminals, from behavioural experiments on trumpet-tailed rats, from measurements of stress hormones in the saliva of children attending daycare centres, and from cohort studies that have tracked the life histories of thousands of individuals for half a century. Burke Harris quotes Dr Robert Block, former president of the American Academy of Pediatrics, as saying 'adverse childhood experiences are the single greatest unaddressed public health threat facing our nation today'. What's true for the United States is almost certainly true for New Zealand – but I believe it won't be 'unaddressed' forever.

I'm proud to have been associated since the early 2000s with Brainwave Trust Aotearoa, which has worked to make sure the latest science – especially research into the effects of trauma on the developing brain – is being heard by those who need to hear it. From prisons to the Beehive, from classrooms to the courts, from hospitals to daycare centres, Brainwave has been spreading the word about the lifelong significance of early childhood experiences, and the changes that could be made to improve outcomes for the adults of the future. In essence, if you can fill the first 1000 days of a child's life with cuddles, attention and kindness, you're setting them up for a happy, healthy and productive adulthood. Get those first 1000 days wrong, and the results are not so great.

The charity was founded in 1998 by New Plymouth paediatrician Dr Robin Fancourt, internationally renowned for her work with abused and neglected children, and author of the book *Brainy Babies*. Robin's interest in this field had been piqued by Texan neurobiologist Bruce Perry's research into the effects of child abuse, and she set up this advocacy charity to spread those ideas further. Early trustees included journalists Sue Younger and Judy Bailey, children's advocate and author Lesley Max, and former principal Youth Court judge Mick Brown, as well a range of others with paediatric, psychological, scientific, legal and business expertise. This mix of qualified people with varying skills working towards the same goal, rather than in their own silos, is what makes Brainwave unique. I was asked to be a trustee because Robin's health was failing and they needed another paediatrician on board. Sadly, Robin died in 2009 of a brain tumour, but the charity she started has gone from strength to strength.

At the outset, Brainwave's activity was focused on trustees like Robin and, later, me, delivering talks about the science to selected groups including Youth Court judges, medical organisations, health visitors, Plunket nurses and play therapists. Meanwhile, Sue and Judy worked to raise public awareness by arranging coverage in newspapers and on TV.

Later, as we attracted generous grants from family endowments and funding trusts, we were able to expand our reach. We sent out our educators into schools and prisons to talk about parenting and brain development, always ensuring that even the most complex of material was made fun and engaging with videos, interactive games and case studies. A recent Brainwave-backed parenting programme for inmates at Christchurch Women's Prison, where 90 per cent of the 130-odd inmates are mothers, focused on strategies for breaking the cycle of family dysfunction. The message of hope here is that there are ways to be an effective parent even if your own childhood was blighted by trauma.

The broad mission has remained the same since Robin founded Brainwave, but in some ways the central goal – of convincing people to take heed of the science – has become easier over time.

Early on, I remember saying to Robin that I'd need some really robust data when presenting to an audience of medical people, because these were evidence-obsessed people who wouldn't settle for a few touchy-feely assertions about the benefits of cuddling children.

To this, Robin would say, 'Well if you want evidence, just read the newspaper.' And sure enough, if you look at someone who's committed a horrible crime at the age of 16, then look at their background, you'll likely see that they've been to five different schools, that they've been forced to witness family violence, that they've been abused themselves. Clearly, said Robin, that person is now wired up in a way that makes them strongly predisposed to violent activity themselves.

This was persuasive but not exactly proof. So it has been gratifying that with each passing year new research is published that supports the contention that these cycles of intergenerational violence are happening because trauma modifies early brain development. It's not only that a child 'learns' to be violent or abusive because that's what they see in their home; there are actual biological changes in their brain and body which create the ideal conditions for them to recreate that dysfunction in the next generation.

HOW BRAINS GROW

To understand how events from childhood might have lifelong effects on a person's brain and overall health, it helps to have a rough idea of how the brain grows during gestation and early childhood.

Within a few weeks of conception, the neurons (nerve cells) in the foetal brain are replicating at a mind-boggling rate, racing towards a final target of around 100 billion cells. Early on the neurons are undifferentiated, but over time they migrate to specific regions of the brain and start to specialise in their function. By around 24 weeks' gestation, all 100 billion cells are in place.

Just because you have 100 billion neurons in position, however, doesn't mean you've got a fully functioning brain yet. Brain activity depends on the network of connections (called synapses) that are made between neurons, and it takes time for neurons to hook up those connections (a process called synaptogenesis). The dramatic increase in brain size that continues after 24 weeks and into the first few years of childhood is due almost entirely to the growth of these new synaptic connections, as well as the reinforcing of existing connections in a process called myelination.

At the time of birth, just 15 per cent of neurons have made any connections – which is more than enough for the new baby to run the basic functions such as breathing, heart rate and blood pressure. After birth, though, there's another explosion in neural connectivity – a period known, charmingly, as 'exuberant synaptogenesis'. All those exuberant neurons are a bit indiscriminate, though, about which other neurons they hook up with; so alongside the synaptogenesis there's an opposite process at work, called 'pruning', where unnecessary and unused synapses are eliminated.

One analogy suggests that you imagine a city full of new buildings (neurons), where some crazy developer has randomly built roads (synapses) between buildings with no plan or organisation.

Some houses end up with 15 roads coming to them, some have two and some have none. As a result, most routes are unwanted, and over time those roads become overgrown or are torn up, while the most useful roads are regularly maintained and widened (myelination). The end result is a city with an orderly transport system that in fact arose from a spate of reckless road-building and a huge amount of tidying up.

It's through these processes of synaptogenesis, pruning and myelination that a young child's brain is first built up, then sculpted into shape. And the sculptor is the environment in which they live. In other words, you get the brain you need for the environment you find yourself in at the time.

A child is born into a bath of sensory inputs – touch, vibration, smell and taste, hearing, vision – and the brain is shaped by what arrives through those senses. Synapses that are useful and well used grow stronger; those that are useless or underused are pruned away. Use it or lose it.

So if a baby is held, stroked, cuddled, sung to, talked to, rocked, fed and loved, the synaptogenesis and pruning of the brain will establish the right sort of connections in the hippocampus, the amygdala, the cingulate gyrus and other curiously labelled parts of the brain besides (those three regions are named, respectively, because they resemble a seahorse, an almond and a girdle!)

This is where the importance of trauma comes in, because stressful experiences interrupt that brain sculpting.

When something scary happens – a lion is chasing you, say – your brain registers the threat and triggers a cascade of processes involving the hypothalamus, the pituitary gland and the adrenal glands to release hormones into the body – most notably adrenaline and cortisol. Adrenaline primes you for 'fight or flight' by raising your pulse, blood pressure and alertness; and cortisol triggers numerous helpful body processes, including unlocking the body's reserves of glucose as you sprint from the lion.

Stress in small doses is a great thing. It stimulates us to do what we need to do in life, whether it's outrunning carnivores or taking a chance in our career. But repeated and large amounts of unresolved stress – the kind that a child might experience if there is constant domestic violence in their household, say – is a different matter.

That's because cortisol, although it's essential to the normal functioning of the body, starts to cause trouble if there's too much of it about. It interferes, at a biochemical level, with the processes of synaptogenesis, myelination and pruning, thus affecting both memory and learning. It can temporarily weaken the immune system, reduce bone density, cause muscles to waste, and leave you with excess blood glucose. The stuff is, frankly, dynamite. In this high-cortisol environment the brain will keep making the connections it needs for short-term survival, but the longer-term consequences of this modified brain wiring can be a problem.

The CDC–Kaiser ACE research is not the only study to show connections between childhood trauma and bad adult outcomes. New Zealand is home to a number of world-renowned longitudinal studies, including the Dunedin Multidisciplinary Health & Development Study (the 'Dunedin Study') and the Christchurch Health & Development Study (the 'Christchurch Study'), both of which have been tracking more than 1000 people from birth since the 1970s, and the Growing Up in New Zealand Study, which started in 2008.

These studies have shown that the markers of a tough childhood are identifiable at birth, and include having a mother who is young, or is a solo parent, or has had numerous partners, or has drug or alcohol problems or a history of psychiatric disease, or an absence of social support. Up until recently the research has focused on the mothers but more recent literature aims to examine both parents in acknowledgement of the role fathers play in child development. The most severe problems occur when there is major disruption of the secure 'attachment relationship' that should form early on between a child and one or more caregivers. Most attachments are formed by six or seven months – the age at which 'stranger anxiety' develops – but the process continues throughout the first couple of years.

Attachment is what underpins a child's ongoing ability to form relationships throughout life. It happens as the adult caregiver carries out simple, repetitive caring actions such as changing a nappy, feeding or playing with their baby. In doing so, both the caregiver and the baby gain pleasure and enjoyment in each other's company and a relationship develops that is warm and nurturing. The American developmental psychologist Urie Bronfenbrenner put it this way: for a child to develop normally, 'somebody has to be crazy about that kid'. This might be someone outside the immediate family – a grandparent, an aunt or a family friend.

The lack of a secure attachment relationship, on the other hand, has been linked to negative outcomes, including high suicide rates and remorseless criminal behaviour.

What is both fascinating and frightening is that attachment (or the lack of it) causes specific structural changes in the brain. In the past decade researchers have looked at the link between parental attachment and brain growth in the South American trumpet-tailed rat, *Octagus degu,* a species whose newborn pups form strong attachment relationships with both father and mother. When researchers separated pups from their parents and later dissected their brains, they found the enforced neglect had wreaked havoc on the physical structures of the brain.

Some brain areas had a deficit of synapses and myelination, while other parts had too many synapses, suggesting that pruning had been interrupted. The mechanisms in rats and humans may not be identical, but we know for certain that when children grow up in an environment of neglect or excessive stress, their brains end up in worse shape.

Research from the burgeoning field of epigenetics – the study of how genes can be switched on or off in an individual by environmental factors – gives some hints about the mechanisms behind this.

In early 2004, American researcher Michael Meaney published a study of rat parenting styles. Mother rats nurture their pups with 'licking and grooming' behaviours, but the extent to which they lick and groom varies widely. Pups raised by highly nurturing mothers tend to become calm adults that don't startle easily, while those who receive little or no nurturing are much more anxious and aggressive as adults. These calmer adults also go on to be more enthusiastic lickers and groomers of their own pups. By swapping pups between mothers, Meaney showed that the differences in adult behaviour were because of the licking and grooming rather than classic Mendelian inheritance. Meaney then showed that the differences in behaviour between the calm and the anxious adults were because their bodies processed cortisol differently. But the really remarkable findings came once he dissected the rats and looked inside their cells. He discovered the altered cortisol-processing was because certain genes had been switched either on or off, causing persistent cellular changes. In other words, licking and grooming (or the absence thereof) was causing epigenetic changes that would last through the rat's lifetime.

In a sense, there's nothing 'bad' about a rat growing up twitchy and aggressive: being ready to respond quickly and strongly to stress is a good survival strategy if your environment is hostile. A rat whose early experiences suggest they're entering a hostile world is simply growing the brain it needs: one that is wired up for 'survival mode'.

It's reasonable to believe the same thing happens in humans. Children who are neglected when young are more likely to become aggressive adults and neglectful parents themselves – not because they've learnt or inherited those behaviours but because their brains and bodies have been epigenetically programmed, at a biochemical level, to respond to stress in a particular way.

There was some heartening news in Meaney's findings, though. He showed that even if a rat pup had been undergroomed and the genetic switches for adult anxiety and aggression were flicked on, it was possible to reverse that process with large doses of remedial licking and grooming, as long as you put the pup back young enough with a super-nurturing mother. In other words, no parent – rat or human – needs to be perfect all the time. Which is very nice to know if you're a parent who's having a bad day.

TEACHING MEN TO BE TENDER

During my twenties I lived in Italy for six months, where I noticed that, as in much of Europe, the elderly and the very young were an integral part of community life. Whether you were eating out, walking in the evening passeggiata or just going about your business, children of all ages, and Nonna and Papa, were there too. This felt very different to the British colonial attitude that 'children should be seen and not heard' and that the elderly should be bundled off to a rest home somewhere out of sight.

I noticed, too, that in Italy men seemed much more likely to kiss and cuddle their children, something I had barely witnessed in the macho New Zealand society of the 1960s and '70s.

Once I'd settled back in New Zealand in the 1980s and was working as a paediatrician, I came to realise this is a real deficit in New Zealand society. We don't teach young men now to be tender and caring and loving. It's not regarded as manly to cry or show emotions or cuddle a baby.

I remember being surprised once when visiting a new baby on the ward to find him surrounded by four tall young men all cooing and cuddling him and expressing protective views about their roles as uncles. The young men were Croatians: here was another European culture that was getting much closer to the ideal of how men should be with their babies.

Too many New Zealand men feel they would appear weak if they were to express affection for a child or take part in the more intimate aspects of child rearing, such as comforting them when they are distressed or sad. I think it's not a coincidence that ours is also a country with one of the highest rates in the OECD of child death from non-accidental injury. Whenever I overhear a father telling a child to 'harden up', it makes me cringe. Gradually the modern New Zealand dad is learning how to relate to his newborn baby, but we have a long way to go. It is interesting to note, too, that fathers tend to offer their children a different type of nurturing experience – they are more likely to engage sons and daughters in rough-and-tumble play and to encourage more risk-taking than mothers are. This type of parenting is complementary to the nurturing and supporting experience typically offered by mothers.

One of the goals of Brainwave's work in schools and in prisons is to make young people aware of what it takes for babies to grow their brains successfully, and to explain the importance of being tender. We want to start early. In many of the Year 11 classes we visit we come across students who are already parents, and many students who are regularly taking care of younger siblings.

Brainwave is making headway on this. Slowly but surely, policymakers and the public are beginning to understand the significance of the first 1000 days of a child's life, and why ensuring a warm and nurturing environment for every child isn't just morally right, but socially and economically sensible.

In Canada, the social entrepreneur Mary Gordon pioneered a programme called Roots of Empathy, where a baby is taken into a classroom of eight- and nine-year-olds for a full day every three weeks, over the course of a year, along with a trainer who leads the class and teacher through an educational programme. The idea is that by seeing the baby close up and tracking their progress from rolling to sitting up to crawling, the pupils develop empathy. They also learn about the rudiments of child brain development, and how to create a safe and nurturing environment for a baby. Meanwhile, the usual subjects – social studies, art, maths and science – are all tweaked to make the baby the focus of interest.

The head teacher at one of the schools told Gordon a lovely story. The teacher had collected a baby from their mother and was carrying it down the corridor to the classroom when she saw two nine-year-old boys fighting in the corridor. They quickly stopped fighting as she came into sight, and she overheard one of them say to the other, 'We'd better stop. Here comes a baby.'

She asked them: 'Why did you say that? I'm the headmistress, so I thought you would have said, "Here comes the headmistress."'

The boy replied, 'Well, we've learnt that you should never fight in front of a baby.'

THE TEENAGE BRAIN: UNDER CONSTRUCTION

At around the age of nine or 10, children begin another burst of synaptic growth and pruning. It's a time when children make a big leap in maturity. Self-centred, wilful behaviours start to be replaced with better impulse control and problem-solving skills, as well as thoughtful decision-making, as the prefrontal cortex – the region just above your eyes and behind your forehead – is remodelled and starts to take the upper hand.

At the same time, the reward centres of the brain – the bits that say 'Just do it! It'll feel good!' – become more sensitive during adolescence. At times it's as if there's a power struggle between the two brain regions – one thoughtful and considered, the other impulsive and pleasure-seeking. Studies have shown that teenagers understand risk as well as any adult, but they're still more likely to indulge in risky behaviours – partly because they figure the reward outweighs the risk, but also because adolescence is a time when peer pressure becomes incredibly important.

This activity in the brain is not helped by the hormonal surges that are fuelling behaviour in the adolescent. They are also trying to work out who they are – what their moral standards are, what sort of adult they will become, what their sexual identity is, what their career plans might be – while at the same time separating themselves from their parents. No wonder they're confused.

Add this all up, and you can only conclude that teenagers are a neurological work in progress, and should be treated a little differently from adults. They are capable of thinking rationally and making sound judgements, but they can't be relied on to do so consistently.

One experiment that demonstrates the way the brain's function changes over the adolescent years involved testing people on their ability to read the emotions in photographs of faces – sad, happy, surprised and so on. The study showed that the older the child, the more accurately they could spot the emotions; and MRI and PET brain scans of the test subjects showed that the part of the brain used for this face recognition was actually shifting with age. Pre-adolescents were using their amygdala – the emotional seat of the brain, while adolescents and post-adolescents were starting to use the prefrontal cortex.

In 2007, in a speech I made on behalf of Brainwave to a conference on youth offending, I pointed out that the pruning in young women's brains is still going strong until they're about 18, and in young men it continues into their early twenties. This, I said, should be taken into account when we form public policy. I argued that the driving age should be raised to 18 and I also supported the then principal Youth Court judge, Andrew Becroft, who said he wanted to see the age of adult criminal responsibility lifted from 17 to 18.

I'm glad to say that the age of driving has shifted up a little (you now have to wait until 16 before applying for a learner's licence), and in late 2016 it was announced that the youth justice age would rise to 18 by 2019 – though this will apply only to low-level crimes; serious violent crimes will still earn automatic inclusion in the adult court system.

SCREEN TIME AND THE BRAIN

The work I've done with my Brainwave hat on has, naturally, had an impact on my paediatric practice.

I had long taken a dim view of the impact of television on children, especially very young children, but a lot of that was based on an intuition (probably connected to having grown up on a farm) that it was a pity for a child to be stuck inside with the curtains drawn when they could be outside climbing trees or making dams in creeks. The real world is a full-throttle multisensory experience: you feel the grass under your feet, hear the birds, smell the air, see the sun and experience the movement of your body through space as you leap into a swimming hole. When you're watching a screen you're using just two senses: vision and hearing. Surely that's an inferior, less enriching experience.

When we looked into this more closely for Brainwave, however, we found a wealth of research to back this intuition. Children who watch a lot of TV spend less time than their peers having conversations with their parents. Big TV watchers have a smaller vocabulary than other children, and spend less time in free play. TV watching in adolescents has been associated with a reduction in exercise and an increase in obesity. Even once the TV's off, the harm persists: big TV watchers have been shown to have more trouble with concentration, and one study showed that they were less inventive in their play. It has also been argued that watching a lot of violence on TV somehow desensitises you to violence, though the evidence on this isn't entirely clear.

Being anti-TV is hardly a radical view: the official stance of the American Academy of Pediatrics is that the right level of screen-time before 18 months is zero (apart from video chatting to communicate with family and friends). For children up to the age of five the academy recommends a maximum of an hour a day and suggests that this should always be with a 'co-viewing' parent who can help them discuss and understand what they're seeing. There is, no doubt, quite some distance between this aspiration and the reality of many children's TV viewing.

The rise of the internet, and social media in particular, makes it much harder than it used to be for parents to draw the line. Most research is clear about the harm of too much passive viewing of an old-school TV broadcast or DVD. Much less is known about the impact on children of the smartphones, tablets, smart TVs and computers that have quite suddenly inserted themselves into every facet of modern life.

It seems likely to me that two-way conversations via a screen – Skyping the grandparents, say – is harmless, seeing as there is a fully interactive human relationship going on. Platforms such as Facebook or Instagram, however, are much murkier, as real interactions with friends overlap with passive consumption of news items, cat videos and mindless clickbait, all delivered in a format that's designed to be ferociously addictive (a quite separate matter that's all about brain chemistry).

Until more research on all this starts to arrive, I would firmly recommend that parents and caregivers try to delay screen time for toddlers for as long as possible, especially under the age of two. Companies that claim to deliver 'educational' games and videos for young children should be treated with particular scepticism. In 2003 it was estimated that a quarter of US households had copies of the 'Baby Einstein' videos, which were marketed as 'educational' for under twos – the very group that shouldn't have been watching TV at all. In 2006 the company, by then owned by Disney, quietly removed all the claims of educational benefits from the marketing, and in 2009 offered full refunds for returned videos, after threats of a class-action lawsuit.

THE 'GOOD ENOUGH' PARENT

For a parent who's already trying to do their best, the Brainwave message can seem a little alarming. Who knew there were so many ways you could ruin your child's future? Fortunately the science also contains some reassuring messages. Yes, it is possible to mess up a child's early years by exposing them to neglect and abuse, but children are pretty resilient, and minor or infrequent falls from parental perfection hardly matter at all.

To count as trauma, the shortfalls have to be quite bad and repeatedly bad. There's no need to beat yourself up because you've come up short on a few occasions.

It's not neglect if your child comes to you with their latest in a series of 20 fingerpaintings when you're tired and just home from work and wanting to sit down and watch TV or read the paper or have a beer, so you don't pay much attention and you're a bit grouchier than you should have been. As long as you're there and give them attention *most* times they ask for it, that's fine.

It's not child abuse if you're exhausted and your young child ends up watching TV all day, just that once.

You haven't destroyed your child's future brain development or put them at risk of mental illness or cardiovascular disease from 'adverse childhood events' because you lost your temper and shouted at your partner in front of them that one time.

There are certain minimum requirements that need to be met for a child to grow up happy and well nurtured, but those minimum standards are not impossibly high, and they're fairly easy to understand. So alongside the warnings about adverse childhood experiences and the like, at Brainwave we also talk about the concept of 'good enough' parenting. In order to thrive and reach their potential, a child doesn't need a super-parent. All they need is a parent who is 'good enough'.

In the case of a newborn baby, that means someone who is taking responsibility for them and is always available: someone who'll feed them when they're hungry, cuddle them when they're sad, change their nappies when they're wet and dirty, and talk to them when they want company. It's hard work, but if you're doing your best most of the time, you're probably doing fine.

A parent's ability to do all this depends quite a lot on how they've been parented themselves, but even someone who has had a difficult childhood can take steps, and be supported, towards ensuring that their child doesn't suffer the same fate.

One rather startling demonstration of 'good enough' parenting arose from an experiment conducted in an Ohio state institution in the 1930s with a cohort of 'orphans' (most were actually abandoned illegitimate babies). Two girls under 18 months who were deemed 'hopeless cases', and whose IQs had been measured as 35 and 46, were transferred for reasons of space to a nearby home for the mentally disabled. There they were placed in a ward for adult women who had a mental age of between five and nine.

When the girls arrived, they were 'pitiful little creatures [who were] emaciated, undersized, and lacked muscle tone or responsiveness. Sad and inactive, the two spent their days rocking and whining.' But when the orphanage psychologist, Harold Skeels, visited six months later, he didn't recognise the girls: their appearance was transformed and their IQs had jumped to 77 and 87. A few months later the scores were remeasured as being in the mid-90s.

When he set about figuring out what had gone so right, Skeels learnt that the girls had received an unusual amount of attention. Ward attendants had bought them toys and books and a couple of the older women had 'adopted' a girl each, showering them with love and affection while the rest of the inmates had acted as 'adoring aunts'.

Intrigued, Skeels devised an experiment. Thirteen more children – all of whom had been assessed as 'mentally retarded' and thus ineligible for adoption – were each placed in the one-to-one care of a mentally disabled teenage girl at the institution. The teenage girls received basic lessons in how to hold, feed, talk to and stimulate their 'baby'. When the babies were transferred, they had an average IQ of 64.

After a couple of years of being mothered and showered with attention by the girls, the babies were changed beyond recognition. Their IQ had leapt by an average 27.5 points, and 11 of the 13 were now considered eligible for adoption to good homes. Over the same period, an unfortunate cohort of 12 similar babies who'd been left back in the normal conditions of the orphanage had suffered an average *fall* in IQ of 26 points.

Twenty-five years later Skeels tracked down the original subjects, and found the 13 transferred children had almost all gone on to lead successful, normal lives, with four of them achieving tertiary qualifications. Meanwhile the 12 who had remained in the orphanage had done far worse: four were still institutionalised, and seven of the remaining eight were working as unskilled labourers.

There are many disturbing things going on at once in this story. What, for instance, happened to those poor teenage girls who became surrogate mothers for a couple of years then had their 'baby' torn away from them? What about the birth mothers, who were more than likely forced to give up their babies because they were unmarried? And what a tragedy that untold thousands of other children in orphanages of the time must have been inflicted with profound mental disability by being starved of cuddles and attention. The parallels with the Romanian orphanages that shocked the world in the late 1980s are obvious.

But the story also proves a point: even these unskilled, uneducated, mentally disabled teenage girls were capable of being perfectly good parents, because all that's really needed to be a 'good enough' parent is time, attention, and a little love.

WHAT ABOUT CHILDCARE?

Time after time, at a Brainwave event or presentation, someone will ask 'What about childcare?' It's a good question. If those first 1000 days are so vital for a child's brain development but both parents (or the sole parent) have to be at work, is it OK to hire strangers to provide all the attention and cuddles and love that we know a child needs for successful brain development?

Other questions arise, too: How do I know if my child's daycare centre is good enough? Is it OK if a caregiver has multiple children to look after? Is a nanny better than a preschool? When is the best time to go back to work? How many hours of childcare outside the family is too much?

Brainwave conducted a comprehensive literature review in 2015 of the available research on the pros and cons of childcare, and the answers are, I'm afraid, messy.

Childcare is an issue where socioeconomic issues, workforce issues, gender issues, neuroscience, politics and parenting all come together in a big complicated knot. Some people don't want to put their children into childcare at all, but have to so they can work. Others want to, but can't afford the quality of childcare they want. Others are perfectly happy with using childcare and feel attacked, or suspect sexism or snobbery, when they're told that it may not be the best thing for their child.

As for the science, before you can say whether childcare is good, bad or neutral, you need to know something about the level of training of the daycare staff, the amount of time a child spends there, the amount of one-to-one time, the age of the child and even, arguably, the sex of the child (boys do slightly less well in childcare than girls).

Or, as Sue Younger and Keryn O'Neill succinctly put it in a summary of the Brainwave literature review: 'It depends.'

There is one important piece of research about childcare that does give me pause, though, given what we know about brain development and the role of stress. In 2004 Australian researcher Megan Gunnar published the results of a study where she took a close look at the cortisol levels in children – conveniently, cortisol levels can be assessed via a quick and simple saliva test – and found that they were consistently higher during the hours the children spent at a daycare centre compared with a similar day at home. As children got older the elevation in cortisol levels became less significant, but for children under two it was almost universal. This research is cause, at the very least, for caution about the risks of daycare for the very young. (If you want to see the nitty gritty of the Brainwave literature review, it's on our website, www.brainwave.org.nz.)

One of the problems in interpreting the research is: How much is too much childcare, and what constitutes good-quality daycare? Government initiatives to increase women in the work force have overemphasised the benefits of early childhood education. They have used research literature that shows that

African-American children in very deprived homes have benefitted from being placed in preschools where parents have also received training. This is not the same as New Zealand children in ordinary preschools. On the other hand, early childhood education is essential in the modern world so we need to make sure that it is of the highest quality.

There was another important limitation in the research we considered: widespread placement of babies and infants in childcare is such a recent phenomenon that solid research about the effect on under-twos is still scarce.

If pressed for a brief answer, I usually say the research – and my experience – suggests that a child is best off spending at least the first year after birth in a close, one-to-one relationship with one or two primary caregivers. If both parents need to be back at work before that year is over, they should delay it as long as they can afford to. Then, if their child is in paid care, the ideal is high-quality childcare, a nanny, or someone trustworthy to establish a good one-to-one relationship with the child.

I think it's crazy that we live in a society that pays people to look after other people's children, yet seems reluctant to pay parents to look after their own. In more enlightened countries such as Sweden, parents get up to two years of paid parental leave to share between them however they like, and most of that is paid at 80 per cent of full salary. The recent announcement that New Zealand is moving to 26 weeks paid parental leave is a step in the right direction, but we're still way behind where we need to be.

This matters because the research shows that putting a child into childcare before they are a year old – especially for long hours – is associated with some negative outcomes, including aggression and other negative behaviour. In certain extreme situations it could even put the attachment relationship with parents at risk.

Once children are a little older, I think childcare is a great option. Apart from anything else, children are social creatures; they need to get out and meet people. They are polishing up their newly developed relationship skills with their peers in a safe environment and, to be honest, by the time they are two and a half to three most of them really love preschool.

A common misconception is that early childhood education is about learning to read and write and count. Preschool education is really about play and relationships and learning how we operate in the social world. Preschoolers are little scientists, constantly exploring the world through play and developing emotional literacy, too – pouring water out of a jug and seeing how much is left, climbing a rope ladder, playing pretend shop with a mate, singing along with friends in a group. There is plenty of time to learn numbers and writing once they're at school.

There's one other reason why you might want to have one parent home for that first year. This might just be the paediatrician in me talking, but it always seems sad when your child takes their first step or says their first word (or their 1000th word for that matter) and it's a stranger who witnesses this rather than a parent.

Wherever this discussion about childcare leads to, most of us as parents will feel conflicted about our choices and wonder whether we are doing or have done the right thing. Often there is no right answer. Fortunately, as stated previously, children are resilient creatures and most of the time things turn out well.

***

Brainwave has partially achieved its goal of getting the message out about the importance of a child's experiences in their early years in determining their future. Some of this success has been through education about the neurobiology of brain development, and some has come about through lobbying politicans and people with influence. I see my work with Brainwave as part of my overall role as a paediatrician in advocating for children, but it has also been personally rewarding and is something I am glad to be involved with.

It's impossible to talk about ideas such as neglect or adverse childhood experiences or childhood trauma without acknowledging the importance of poverty in our society. More than 200,000 children are living in poverty in New Zealand – meaning that they are missing out on warm clothing, access to healthcare, adequate housing and good nutrition. They are at a heightened risk of chronic illness, of child abuse and neglect.

Being poor doesn't automatically mean there will be abused and neglected children, but it does add huge stresses to a person's life, some of which can translate directly into trauma for the children in a struggling household.

The science of those first 1000 days tells us that every child needs 'good enough' parenting if they are to thrive. A 'good enough' parent for every child doesn't seem a lot to ask, but we're not there yet. And as we've learnt from the newspaper headlines – and as I have sometimes been forced to witness at first-hand through my work in NICU – the consequences when we fall short can be horrifying.

CHAPTER 9

CHILDREN RAISING CHILDREN

Any family you meet in NICU will be under tremendous stress for months, merely because they have a very premature or very unwell child.

They were lovely-looking baby boys. Born at Auckland Hospital at 29 weeks' gestation, they were originally triplets but their sibling had died at birth. They were healthy and reasonably stable, each a little over 1000 grams, and looked likely to do well, though being 10 weeks premature they would still need at least a month of hospital care.

Within days of the babies' birth, their parents got into an ugly shouting match in the corridor and one of them had to be escorted outside. I remember thinking we needed to get the babies transferred as soon as possible to Middlemore NICU, where they would be closer to the support of their wider family in Mangere and Clendon in South Auckland. The family obviously had some social issues – and when parents are experiencing strife, stresses such as finding taxi fares and fighting rush-hour traffic between home and hospital don't help.

The babies were transferred to Middlemore a few days later. I heard nothing more about them until 11 weeks later when I received a message from the paediatric intensive care unit (PICU) next-door at Starship – a courtesy call, really, seeing as these boys had recently been through my unit.

Something shocking had happened. The boys had been admitted a few days earlier and one had just died. Both had traumatic brain injuries – and I later learnt that both had suffered broken ribs in previous incidents. When I went down to the ward the surviving boy, Cris, was lying there on life support. The injuries were sickening, and it was clear he wasn't going to survive. He died that evening, 13 hours after his brother.

Once the media learnt about their violent deaths, their names – Cris and Cru – would become a byword for New Zealand's child abuse epidemic, for the deep dysfunction within some families, and the failure of our state services to protect vulnerable children. These were the 'Kahui twins' – the sons of Chris Kahui and Macsyna King.

Over the coming years there would be a trial and a coronial inquest, countless newspaper articles, TV reports and a 'tellall' book containing implausible theories. We would learn the details of the injuries suffered by the boys, and the apparently uncaring attitudes of his parents and their wider whānau, who should have been looking after two vulnerable premature babies but were instead caught up in chaotic, messy lives characterised by violence and addiction.

We all watched as 12 members of the wider family stonewalled police attempts to find who was responsible for the death, and we recoiled as we learnt some of the details: how Macsyna King was offered a bed in a family room at Starship so she could stay with her dying children but told nurses she didn't 'give a shit' and wanted to get home. How when Chris Kahui was told that his children were gravely ill and he should come in to the hospital, he allegedly hung up the phone and returned to his video game. We heard how Child, Youth and Family removed a one-year-old and a six-month-old from two properties where the twins had lived, and reported that they were neglected, malnourished and dirty. At trial Chris Kahui was found not guilty of murdering his boys, but the 2012 coroner's inquest pointed the finger of blame back at him, stating that the twins' fatal injuries occurred while they were in his 'sole custody, care and control'.

On that day in June 2006, of course, I knew none of this. I knew two babies that had once been in my care had died, almost certainly as a result of non-accidental injuries, and I wanted to know what had happened.

I contacted Lindsay Mildenhall, head of NICU at Middlemore, and asked him what he knew. He told me they had been well aware that the babies were at higher risk than normal, so they'd taken all the appropriate steps to make sure someone was keeping an eye on them after they left the unit. He said the babies had been a good weight and well nourished, and every time the homecare nurses visited everything seemed fine. Freshly laundered bedding and clothes and nappies were piled up next to the cot they shared. 'Everything looked perfect,' Lindsay said. 'We had no idea.'

A decade on, the Kahui case has not lost its power to shock, even though there have been more like it since. Somehow the fact of their being twins (or triplets, as we in the unit continued to think of them) added to the horror; and the fact that no one was ever held accountable for their deaths is hard to stomach. Their deaths have become emblematic of one of the darkest aspects of New Zealand society: the fact that some families have no clue about how to provide the rudiments of care, nurture and physical safety for their children. In the extreme cases the question is not so much whether a child can thrive in such an environment, but whether they can even survive it.

I don't pretend to have the solutions to this large and complex problem, but working in neonatal intensive care in a public hospital (and to a lesser extent my private paediatric work) has at the very least given me some perspectives on the causes and consequences of inadequate parenting.

***

Any family you meet in NICU will be under tremendous stress for months, merely because they have a very premature or very unwell child. There is constant travel between home and hospital to care for the child and for the mother to drop off expressed milk. There will be all sorts of unexpected costs, even though the hospital care is state-funded. The family income may have fallen recently with the mother not working (and, in the case of a prem baby, months earlier than expected). There may be other children at home to care for.

Most parents, most of the time, amaze me as they rise to the challenge, coping with the uncertainty, the setbacks, the struggles of their child and the exhaustion of it all. But under such conditions, tempers fray and tears are seldom far away, even for people who are financially and socially well resourced and in good mental health. So I advise junior staff to be prepared for a certain amount of bad behaviour by parents, and not to take it to heart.

There are limits, though. On a few occasions, after a parent has started swearing or shouting at me or my colleagues, I've taken them aside for a quiet word: 'Please, don't you give me a hard time. I know your baby is sick and he's got major heart and respiratory problems and that's very hard, but I didn't cause that. I'm here to help you. Just because that's happening to your baby is no excuse for you to be rude to me or my staff in that way.' Usually, after the initial shock when they realise they're being told off, they look a bit mortified, mutter a quick 'Sorry', and settle right down.

When someone is acting in a seriously threatening way, anyone on staff can dial a special code that triggers a 'code orange', and security staff rush to the scene to restrain the culprit or escort them off the premises. (Once upon a time hospitals didn't need to bother with such things, but after a baby was 'stolen' from Middlemore many years ago, security protocols were instigated – including door entry codes and monitored access.)

We had to call a code orange the time a father came into NICU, pushed his way past a couple of nurses and lifted his baby out of his incubator, then headed for the exit. His child was far too young to survive for long without NICU resources, so he had to be stopped.

The father was an intimidating figure, rough-looking and solidly built and, we discovered later, with prison time under his belt, but as we waited for the security staff to arrive I managed to get between him and the exit and engage him in conversation. 'Look,' I said to him, 'let's not stand here in the middle of the unit getting in everyone's way. Let's go and have a chat.'

In a side room he told me he was estranged from the mother and felt that the family's social worker had it in for him. He was extremely unhappy that he wasn't getting any access to his baby, as he had a genuine desire to be a real dad, which was why he'd come to take him home.

I said, 'OK, I know how you feel. You've had a baby and it looks like you're not going to get enough access. We can work towards making that possible for you, but it will become completely impossible if you walk out that door with your baby.'

I said he should let us have the baby so we could look after him, and I told him I would arrange for our social workers to look at making a plan where he could come and see his baby when he wanted. To my relief, he succumbed like a lamb and handed the baby over. I kept up my end of the bargain, requesting that visiting arrangements be made for him, but later the situation deteriorated and he was 'trespassed' from the hospital. He had had an abusive and neglectful upbringing himself, and had no idea of how to behave in these environments. All the same, the safety of our staff had to come first, and I was acutely aware of how frightening the experience had been for the two nurses.

I felt real sympathy with this man, and I feel it for others like him. The world of babies is one populated by midwives and Plunket nurses and health visitors and early childhood education teachers, almost all of whom are women. Men can end up feeling sidelined.

In the case of this would-be kidnapper, one might argue that he *deserved* to be sidelined, but even fathers who are doing everything right sometimes feel excluded from early parenting. You could attribute this to the persistence of traditional gender roles and the fact that fathers are more likely than mothers to be back at work in the early months. But there are other factors at play, too. There is good research, for example, showing that in neonatal units, including ours, staff mostly talk to the mother rather than the father.

In my experience, the exclusion of fathers is most obvious where a mother who perhaps hasn't had the benefit of a good education or a rewarding career has a baby and finds it's something she's really good at. She's understandably keen to lay claim to an area of expertise that's all her own. So when the father picks up the baby she says, 'Give him to me. You're hopeless with the baby!' and he is shut out and never develops those skills. I'm sure this dynamic is changing for the better – many fathers are both offering and being expected to play a fuller role in their children's early years – but it's still more common than you might think.

It's not only aggressive fathers who try to uplift babies against our advice. Once I had to counsel a mother and grandmother – both of them high on P – from doing the same. I finally got through by reminding them that acting with such disregard for their baby's wellbeing would almost certainly lead to the child being taken away from them by CYF (now MCOT, the Ministry for Children–Oranga Tamariki). Just because people have different ideas about parenting than I do doesn't mean they'll necessarily be bad parents – but use of hard drugs is definitely not on.

A neonatal unit is a window on the world outside, and we have to find ways of coping whenever we brush up against some of the darker realities of that world, whether it's drug-taking, crime, domestic violence or family abuse.

Once, in NICU, a nurse had been asking a mother why she was choosing not to breastfeed, and the mother replied that her brother-in-law had a methamphetamine lab in the basement of the house where she lived, and she was worried about the effect on her baby of ingesting milk that might be contaminated as a result.

We now had the dilemma of whether to include this information about an alleged serious crime in the parental home in the transfer letter to the level 2 unit that the baby was moving to, or whether we should just talk vaguely about 'serious social issues'. We knew from bitter experience that if you disclose such information to police or the MCOT and they take action because of it, you can make things much worse for the mother as she could be identified as a nark.

In the end we fudged things: we left the information out of the file, but we rang the level 2 consultant and let them know informally.

***

As I mentioned earlier, one of my jobs at the hospital is treating babies whose mother has taken opioids such as heroin or methadone during pregnancy – weaning them off a low dose of morphine over several weeks. Drug-addicted mothers come from all walks of life, from the

Remuera mum with the Audi and children in private school to the teen mum with gang associations who's living a chaotic, near-itinerant life. Usually mother and child live together at the hospital, baby's cot beside mum's bed, until the baby is fully weaned off the drug.

One day in the late 1990s I was showing a young registrar how our neonatal drug-withdrawal regimen worked, and gave him the usual spiel about how it was important to suspend judgement about our patients. 'We're paediatricians,' I said, 'so our focus is on the baby. It's not our job to judge the mother or her choices. We need to be impartial and talk to her about the baby's needs, and stay matter-of-fact when asking things that might normally be a bit shocking, like how often she was taking her drug of choice.'

We then walked into the ward to talk to a mother who had been on methadone during pregnancy. We chatted a bit, but then the mother made some complaint about the competence of one of the staff nurses who was looking after her baby, and implied that some of the baby's problems were related to the standard of care rather than the fact that he was going through methadone withdrawal.

Perhaps I'd got out of the wrong side of bed that morning, or I'd seen too many babies already that day wriggling with discomfort and wailing with the characteristically incessant and high-pitched cry of a drug-withdrawing neonate.

Whatever the reason, I blew a fuse and launched into a 30-second rant. 'How *dare* you criticise our staff,' I raged. 'You've put your baby in jeopardy by taking drugs that your baby is now withdrawing from. You've endangered his life and health and made his life a misery. And yet you're suggesting it's not your fault, and *we're* to blame? Well we're not. I wonder if awful people like you should be allowed to have children at all!'

I then stormed out, not especially keen to hear her reaction.

Moments later I turned to my protégé and said, somewhat sheepishly, 'So, that's precisely what you must never, *ever* do when dealing with these mothers. Don't let them get under your skin.'

It was a pretty bad lapse of professionalism on my part, and one the registrar wickedly recounted during his leaving speech when he left Auckland to become medical director of a major Australian neonatal unit. But over the years I have, by and large, *not* let them get under my skin.

I know that some of the parents we see in NICU who aren't behaving well have usually had impossibly difficult childhoods of their own. And as I know from my work with Brainwave, it's extraordinarily tough to overcome the emotional baggage and developmental deficits that were installed all those years earlier.

I also have to remember that I'm seeing a statistically skewed population of parents. In

NICU we see a disproportionately large number of parents who are underprivileged, because it turns out that being underprivileged is *in itself* a strongly causal factor for having a premature baby.

In this following example I've freely merged elements of numerous cases to avoid identifying anyone in particular, but here is the kind of situation we encounter.

A 17-year-old girl from one of the poorer parts of Northland, who is already known to social agencies because of a multigenerational history of wider family dysfunction, has gone through early pregnancy without receiving any antenatal care. When she starts to get frequent headaches at around 18 weeks, caused by pregnancy-related high blood pressure, she doesn't know it's a problem and there's no one around who knows enough to tell her otherwise.

The high blood pressure continues, causing growth restriction and impaired blood supply to the foetus, along with a constellation of other problems. If she had attended antenatal classes she would have been given information about the adverse effects of alcohol on her unborn baby, but instead she drinks throughout the pregnancy, including a number of binge events. She smokes. She eats a lot of junk food, not aware that the resulting excessive weight gain increases the risk of gestational diabetes. She has bacterial vaginosis, an imbalance of bacteria in the vagina which increases the risk of miscarriage or premature birth.

The net effect is that at 27 weeks she develops pre-eclampsia and goes into labour. In an ideal world she would be delivering the baby in a big city hospital such as Auckland where the highest-level intensive care would be immediately available for her baby. But she lives in a far from ideal world; she arrives at her local hospital so close to delivery that a transfer by air ambulance has to wait until after the birth. Postnatal transfers are associated with worse outcomes than antenatal transfers, but in this case there was no time.

The father is 18, and because of his history of violence in a previous relationship the mother is not allowed any contact with him now she's having a child. If he's around her, the child is liable to be removed from her custody by social workers. Or perhaps the father is relatively blameless and can be involved in parenting his premature child, but is young and from a tough background, and he's immature. When he comes in to the NICU he feels out of his depth and makes up for it with bluster and swagger and a combative bluntness with staff.

Both parents are doing their best and we're doing our best, but we are watching as they handle the baby in the unit and as they interact with each other, and we're wondering: Are these child-parents really going to be able to take care of their child?

Over the months that the baby is in our care, relatives from the wider family come along to offer support but, instead, spend their time picking fights with the mother and the clinical staff. We tend to forget that when a baby is sick or premature it is not only the parents who suffer. The grandparents suffer twice over: anxiety about the baby but also anxiety and heartache for their own babies – the parents. Often their own obstetric and parental traumas are re-ignited and cause them to react in ways that are not always helpful for parents or staff.

Three months later, we have successfully 'rescued' the 17-year-old's baby from the perils of extreme prematurity. There's been a gut surgery for necrotising enterocolitis, laser treatment for oxygen-related retinopathy, and he has developed chronic lung disease and will need a home oxygen supply for several months – but the child is ready, in a medical sense at least, to be discharged to the home. The parents have by now moved permanently to the Auckland area, where they have more whānau support and can be closer to the baby.

Yet the behaviour we've seen from the parents and their families doesn't fill us with confidence. We pass on our concerns to MCOT, and the social workers and homecare nurses visit the home and meet members of the wider family.

We take some comfort from changes we have observed in the mother over the past four months, due in part to the mentoring and role-modelling our staff have given her. She has come in some days feeling sad and the nurses have comforted her, put an arm around her and shown her the wonderful things her baby is capable of doing. She now knows what a fever means, when to take the baby to the doctor, all about feeding and comforting an unsettled baby. She understands which cries are hunger and which are pain. She herself has been looked after, has seen at firsthand what tender parenting can look like, and has gained a sense of achievement and some maturity.

A discharge plan is developed that includes everything from instructions for using the oxygen correctly, to the names of relatives who've promised to provide social support to the parents. We talk to the parents about infant resuscitation and the best sleeping position to reduce the risk of cot death, and make sure they have the number of a GP they can contact with any small problems.

We try to ease the transition back home by giving the baby and parents a couple of nights in an onsite 'parents room' where they can get used to taking responsibility for their baby on their own, with staff available right next door if they need them.

Everything is in place. All the boxes have been ticked. We discharge the child, but we wave goodbye with a heavy heart because we have a feeling that the 'home' this child is going to is still far from ideal. Our job is done, but we're crossing our fingers that MCOT know what they're doing and have put adequate support in place.

***

Families who have done it tough – some of whom go on to make things tough for us in NICU – are only a fraction of the families who come through the unit. Maybe 5–10 per cent of cases have this sort of flavour, but they consume a lot more of our time and energy, so it feels like more. The vast majority of our families are the exact opposite: resourceful, resilient and kind.

We're always being surprised. Sure, poverty – both material and emotional – has been part of many parents' experience, but they can still find time to thank us for our efforts. Recently the mother of a child who had been with us for weeks phoned from another hospital where they had gone for palliative care, to tell me especially that her daughter had died. She said, 'You were her family and we felt very loved by all of you so I wanted you to know.'

I could hardly contain my tears as I stepped back into our ward meeting to tell everyone. What better reward can you have for just doing your job?

***

The death of the Kahui twins was profoundly depressing for many people, but for NICU staff specifically it was an extreme demonstration of all the things we fear when sending a vulnerable child home.

At the time I thought, 'We have failed so badly here.' I also thought, 'Oh god, why do we even bother?'

It is very easy to be seduced by the glamour and heroism of neonatal intensive care. You put in the lines and tubes and hook up the monitors and machines that breathe on behalf of the baby, and you feel great because you've saved a life, and spent a couple of hundred thousand dollars doing so. But all that is for naught if the child is going home to parents who haven't a clue how to look after a child.

There is a philosophical dilemma I sometimes put to junior staff when teaching: if you had two babies delivered at the same time and you only had one intensive care cot available, which baby would you save by giving them the bed? The baby whose parents had done everything they could to ensure a healthy pregnancy and who looked likely to take care of the baby once discharged? Or the baby whose parents had made unhealthy decisions throughout pregnancy and didn't seem to care what happened to their child? (I'll never forget the mother who, when we sat her down to deliver the sad news that her baby had died while she was out, shrugged and said: 'Yeah, I thought the baby might cark it.')

The juniors always try to wriggle away from the central ethical question by finding a workaround: 'Well, I'd get on the phone and find a bed in Australia', or 'I'd give priority to the baby that was born five seconds earlier.' There is, of course, no good answer to the question, but medical ethics dictate that you must respect the autonomy of each individual baby regardless of the baggage they may arrive with. We do our best not to let our personal feelings about parents cloud our judgement as we treat their child.

My other snap reaction to the Kahui case was that it confirmed all the negative stereotypes I used to hold about some urban Māori – disconnected from their culture and stuck in a rut of welfare benefits, dysfunction, addiction and violence. Those stereotypes had only been reinforced by some of my experiences in NICU. Now I feel ashamed of that reaction, and over the years I've frequently been reminded not to judge a book by its cover.

Some time ago I was looking after a pair of 28-weeker twins in NICU. They were stable and doing fine for their age. But one weekend one of the twins suddenly needed a blood transfusion – something that required parental consent. We tried to find the parents, but they'd disappeared and we had no idea how to contact them as their cellphone was switched off, so we went ahead in the expectation of retrospective consent. This is legally defensible in a life-threatening situation, but it's not the way we like to operate.

It seemed to me that this was another pair of feckless parents from up North who had no sense of responsibility and didn't care what happened to their vulnerable newborn babies. When they returned to the unit on the Monday I sat them down and was about to read them the riot act, explaining what it took to be a good parent. Once they'd told me what had actually happened, though, I felt embarrassed.

The couple had originally dashed down to Auckland because the twins were coming early, and had made only temporary arrangements for their older children back at home in Northland. Those arrangements had recently ended, so they'd had to go home, pick them up and make new arrangements – and they knew their twins were safe with us. Yes, it would have been helpful if they'd told us their plans, but they were in fact being sensible and responsible parents. I apologised and resolved to think twice before jumping to conclusions.

I had a similar moment of clarity in the 1990s when I was making an advice video for parents of prem babies and interviewing parents whose babies were currently in the unit. Our unit's social worker identified those parents who were willing to talk on camera, including a young Māori woman whose 27-weeker was doing pretty well.

I'd not spent much time getting to know the mother in the unit, as she seemed a rather angry individual and slightly intimidating in appearance, right down to the cross tattooed on her forehead. Once she started talking about her experience with her baby, though, I realised she was extremely thoughtful and sensitive. She eloquently articulated the emotional complexities of her situation, and had a calm and spiritual view of what was going on for her and her baby son.

I realised that her apparent negativity and fierceness were a reflection of her distress and possibly shyness rather than anger, and that I'd probably placed too much weight on that tattoo. I kicked myself for having been narrow-minded, and resolved to do better in future.

My thinking shifted again as recently as 2016, when a group of Brainwave's trustees and educators made an extended visit to the Ngāti Toa marae in Wellington. I found the experience truly mind-expanding. Growing up in rural South Otago where the Māori population was small, and coming from mostly Scottish and Irish stock, I'd had virtually no experience of Māori culture apart from some simplistic rose-tinted teachings in school. And despite my many years of working for Māori parents and children, and alongside Māori staff, this marae visit shuffled me sideways into a different and much more sympathetic understanding of the position of Māori in Aotearoa.

There was much discussion on the marae of the Treaty of Waitangi and the injustices dating back to 1840. But for me it was also a moving personal experience. The Ngāti Toa marae looks out to Mana Island, a great slab of bare rock and earth off the coast of Plimmerton: you can sense the importance of place there. In the water you can see stingray wings rippling the water as they swim close to shore, and those same wings are also present in the carvings and weavings of the meeting house where we slept the night and where members of the marae explained to us the significance of the art and craftwork there.

One thing that resonated with me was the Māori practice of relating your origins to place and the land. I, too, feel defined by the lakes, rivers and mountains of my childhood, and much of what speaks to me in my environment makes sense when put into the context of Māori values. I feel I still have a long way to go in this respect. I have done a couple of workshops looking more specifically at how race and culture affect the determinants of health outcomes.

The more I learn, the more I'm inclined to step back and take a broader view of the bad and sad behaviour I see in NICU. I can see that some people are starting 25 metres behind the starting line, and that has to be taken into account. It's not good enough to look at a young woman from a poor Māori family in Northland, who's in her early twenties and onto her fifth or sixth pregnancy and not managing at all well, and just throw up your hands and accept that's the way things are, or to make harsh judgements about her.

Rather, we need to see her struggles and say that we as a society have to do something to support these parents and their children. We have to find a way to circumvent some of the harm. It's important to remember, too, that there are many families of Pākehā or other ethnicities who are also in a bad way; these problems affect Māori disproportionately, but not just Māori.

It's going to be complicated and difficult, but as we consider the causes and the possible cures, we would do well to follow the money and look at the effects of economic inequality. That's exactly what Brainwave did in a recent literature review of research into the effects of child poverty on child development – and what we learnt deserves to be heard more widely. New Zealand is a rich country, but we have a poverty problem.

CHAPTER 10

BREAKING THE CYCLE

In innumerable ways, poverty puts a family under stress and creates an environment less conducive to healthy child development.

My childhood was, without question, idyllic. My brother and I grew up on a busy farm on the banks of the Pomahaka River in South Otago with parents who were loving, interested in our wellbeing and financially comfortable. We had security, but also freedom: long uninterrupted summers swimming in the river or playing in the surf near our rented bach at Kaka Point; biking into the Blue Mountains with friends with picnic lunches packed by our parents; spending hours up in the trees in the pine plantation behind the house.

Our mother had a voracious interest in the world beyond Otago, and always insisted we celebrate all of life's small moments. She once scolded me for not putting my name down to go with a school party to hear Louis Armstrong because it seemed expensive: 'You may only have one chance in life to hear the world's greatest jazz musician – the money is not important.'

Our extended family, most of whom lived in the upper Clutha, was huge – I had more than 40 first cousins, and in summer we'd all meet up in Wanaka or Hawea. We would take off in convoy across the Haast Pass and have huge picnics on the Haast river banks, a swim on the West Coast and arrive back in moonlight, exhausted. Our parents helped show us the breadth of the world, but also showed us that we could take part in it. On Friday evenings we'd all drive 30 miles into Gore – the big smoke – where we'd change our six library books, have a fish and chip dinner at the local grill then go to a movie. I remember on a couple of occasions stopping on the way home and getting out of the car to watch the Southern Lights. The skies were amazing, but the real memories were of our parents making sure that we were experiencing life.

Technically speaking, I wasn't entirely spared all the childhood traumas enumerated in the CDC–Kaiser ACE study, given that my mother was bipolar, and mental illness in a parent is ranked as an 'adverse childhood event'. The times when she became deeply depressed were indeed confusing and sometimes frightening for us children, but I also remember her exuberance and joy when she was on a high. And throughout it all my father kept things on an even keel, so I suspect I was mostly unscarred by the experience.

The point I'm making is that in all the ways that really matter, I had a childhood of extraordinary privilege – not butlers and Rolls Royces and trust funds, but nurture, love, stability and social connection.

Of course I'm hardly alone in this. Many New Zealanders have a great childhood. But far too many don't, and though the reasons for this are complex and many, there is one factor that must not be ignored: the effects of a child of growing up in an environment of poverty.

Since the 1980s, rates of childhood poverty in New Zealand have almost doubled. In 2015,

Brainwave researcher Hilary Nobilo put together an excellent review of what researchers have to say about the connections between poverty and child development, and the findings (which I'm leaning on pretty heavily in this section) are harsh.

Some of the numbers shift from year to year – the exact number of children living in poverty, the quantum of benefit payments, the level of unemployment – but the big picture remains the same: in innumerable ways, poverty puts a family under stress and creates an environment less conducive to healthy child development. And as we already know, the conditions during the first few years of a child's life will echo through their entire life and into the lives of *their* children.

Poverty in New Zealand isn't evenly spread. Māori and Pasifika children are twice as likely as New Zealand European children to be living in severe and persistent poverty. Children living in a solo-parent family will do it tougher – either because there's only one income or because the parent is dependent on benefits that, for many years now, have been set at a level that's technically high enough to live on but low enough to be mildly punitive.

When you live in poverty the problems come from multiple directions at once, and they all compound each other: you're likely to be living in crummy housing that's cold and damp and overcrowded, and this contributes to episodes of ill-health. Your access to healthcare is likely to be compromised: either you can't afford the care, or you can't afford the transport to get there, or you're working in the kind of low-status job where time off to take a child to the doctor is much harder to arrange.

Even something as fundamental to the nation's health as widespread immunisation is compromised by the effects of poverty. Many of the New Zealand children who miss out on immunisation do so not by choice but because they don't have easy access to healthcare. In rural areas of New Zealand especially, we need more resources to ensure that those without the necessary education, or the money for petrol, are assisted in getting their children to clinics. Māori and Pasifika children have lower immunisation rates than Pākehā – and way higher rates of rheumatic fever, impetigo and pneumonia. Much of the infectious disease we see here is the kind of thing you'd expect to see in developing countries, not in a wealthy, developed society such as New Zealand.

Most of my first-hand knowledge of socioeconomic deprivation comes from my work in the public hospital system with newborns and their parents; my private paediatric patients tended to be relatively well off. But from time to time I helped out with older children, too. Once, a midwife told me she'd recently delivered a baby and when she was paying a home visit she saw that the baby's seven-year-old brother had shocking impetigo (school sores) all over his legs. Could I pay a visit and check him out?

The family were Pasifika overstayers so were unable to get him registered with the local GP, and they couldn't really afford to take him to the doctor anyway. I went to the address: a state house in Mt Roskill that was utterly crammed with people – in one bedroom I counted 10 mattresses on the floor. The boy was lying on one and the mother was lying beside him with the baby. The boy had suppurating sores full of pus all over his legs.

Infections can hit anyone, but here the significance of the family's poverty was blindingly obvious: overcrowding in the home increased the chance of impetigo contagion, and poor nutrition possibly meant his immunity was lower. I prescribed the boy some antibiotics, and sent a swab to the lab for analysis. A few days later the results came back showing it was an antibiotic-resistant strain so I switched to another, stronger antibiotic and eventually the infection cleared up. It wasn't a medically complicated situation, but lack of cash and social insecurity meant delayed treatment, unnecessary suffering for the boy, and an increased risk of infection for the many others at the address.

On another occasion I treated a 17-year-old boy who had epilepsy. His parents, too, were overstayers and so although they had found a GP who would see him, referral to public neurological services wasn't possible. He was struggling along completely untreated and had started missing a lot of school because of frequent fits. After I saw him I rang a colleague who was a paediatric neurologist and explained the situation, and he was able to treat him for free – in the end all he needed was long-term prescription of a common epilepsy drug. It was another situation where something relatively manageable had spiralled into a much larger problem because a family was lacking in financial and social resources.

As I know only too well from my experiences in NICU, poverty starts messing with a child's chances long before they're born, given that a mother living in poverty is more likely to have a poor diet, more likely to smoke, more likely to drink, and more likely not to attend antenatal classes. She's also more likely to be experiencing greater day-to-day stress because of financial difficulties or overcrowding, and that stress can have direct effects on foetal development due to various hormonal and chemical signals passed on through the placenta.

Once the child has arrived (and quite aside from the additional burdens if the child is premature), poverty starts interfering with the quality of parenting. Financial pressures alone turn up the stress in a household, and though most parents experiencing poverty don't mistreat their children, research shows that harsh, punitive or inconsistent parenting occurs at higher rates when the family is experiencing poverty. Once again, you can see the potential for some of those adverse childhood events such as physical abuse, which, by affecting brain development and cortisol response, sets a child up for a more difficult, more sickly and less successful adulthood.

Even in a country like New Zealand with a public health system where a lot of treatment is provided free, poverty has a huge impact on physical health. Children from poorer families suffer more infectious diseases and stomach bugs, more respiratory problems and injuries. They have less access to care, and even heavily subsidised part-charges are too much to cover.

Children in poor homes are likely to have fewer books, fewer toys, fewer safe places to play – and with each passing year the bad news accumulates. Children who experience poverty often start school less prepared, meaning that before they've even started their education they're falling behind their better-off peers. Poorer grades, fewer years in school, lower earnings as an adult, and hey presto – another cycle of economic disadvantage underway.

Nobilo's literature review ends on a slightly more positive note, however. The obvious point to make is that being poor doesn't mean all these outcomes are inevitable for a given child: many children who grow up in poverty do fine, and that's usually because they're being protected by some aspects of the parenting they're receiving, especially the healthy attachment relationships that Brainwave likes to talk about.

We need to keep encouraging parents to cuddle and talk to their children and read to them and make them feel loved.

Some big problems will need high-level political and economic decisions if they are to be solved. For example, New Zealand has a scandalously large proportion of cold, inadequate housing. The government that directly addresses the supply and quality of housing – especially rental housing, as that's where poorer people are more likely to live – could make a big difference fast. I was heartened, during the 2017 election campaign, to hear both major parties talking about child poverty and housing standards, and I was even happier to see that the party that I believe is taking these issues more seriously is now leading the coalition govenment.

There's another solution to poverty that's so obvious it sometimes gets overlooked: directly putting more cash into the pockets of the poorest people in our society by tweaking the benefit and taxation systems. There's good research linking children's academic achievement to the size of family income, and the effect is greatest in the child's early years. Again, there's reason to hope that a left-leaning government will be more inclined to see the poorest among us as deserving of compassion and a hand-up, rather than judgement and derision.

***

Another group of parents who struggle with similar issues to those living in poverty are refugees. They face both economic and psychosocial hardship. From the late 1990s we have seen a number of mothers coming through the maternity services who are HIV-positive. This has implications for the health of their baby. If a mother has untreated HIV infection there is an over 25 per cent risk of transfer of the virus to the infant, who is then infected for life. Identifying the mother's status in pregnancy is important because there are measures we can take to reduce the risk for the baby to virtually zero: treating the mother during the pregnancy to suppress the viral load, giving intravenous treatment in labour, and then treating the baby for the first month. Initially it was hard, in New Zealand, to get groups such as Maternity Action to agree to test the mothers. They argued that it was an invasion of the mother's privacy – despite the fact that most mothers would like to ensure that their baby would be protected from the virus if there was any risk. Eventually, after a few years of wrangling we managed to have universal testing for HIV at maternal booking as an opt-out choice.

When we first encountered these HIV-positive mothers they were mostly sub-Saharan African refugees, but over time the range of ethnicity has changed: now about half the mothers are from Africa where HIV infection is endemic, and the rest are New Zealand

European, Asian and Pasifika. In Auckland we have managed and treated over 90 babies – and since 1995 we have had no transmission of HIV from mother to baby. This is despite having some sick mothers, one of whom subsequently died of AIDS, and some extremely preterm babies. I follow the children up in my clinic for two or three years to check on the effects of the medication and, of course, to check for evidence of the virus. In doing so it is rewarding to get to know the families and the trials they have experienced.

I remember one young mother from Rwanda. I discovered while chatting to her at a follow-up clinic that she had been involved in the civil war there, where approximately 800,000 people (70 per cent of the Tutsi population) were killed and hundreds of thousands of women were raped and subsequently developed HIV. She had lost her husband in the fighting, escaped to Uganda and remarried there. She had discovered, when she immigrated to New Zealand, that she was HIV-positive – this was felt to be a death sentence at that time, before current drug treatment was available. All this and she was still only 26. She always turned up at clinic beautifully presented with her gorgeous child, who is doing well. I could only marvel at what some people experience in life and that they still remain positive.

***

I'm not a politician or an economist, but in the area where I have a little experience – the public health system – I sometimes shake my head at the folly of reforms that are justified on the grounds of 'rationalisation' or 'efficiency' but look suspiciously like cost-cutting and corner-cutting.

In 1984 the reforming Labour government gave New Zealand's health system a huge shove in the direction of a 'market' approach. Managers and accountants with corporate experience descended on the health sector in swarms and told us to start thinking of ourselves as business units. Doctors who had previously focused on patients were expected to spend much more time on budgets and reports and 'job-sizing' exercises.

It's arguable that some changes were positive, but it was often hard to tell amid the chaos as successive health ministers unleashed wave after wave of structural changes. Health boards were amalgamated then separated then amalgamated again; hospitals were encouraged to compete with each other, undermining the collegiality between clinicians in different locations; hospital user charges were introduced, then dropped because of public outcry. Clinicians like me seethed through long meetings chaired by managers who didn't know one end of a scalpel from the other, as they explained to us how medicine should be done.

Mostly, we gritted our teeth and soldiered on, but there were a few specific changes that I found especially disappointing – including what's known as 'early maternal discharge': the policy of getting mothers to go home as soon as possible after a hospital birth.

It was once common for a mother to stay in hospital for a week or even two after giving birth, during which time she'd be fed, looked after and supported in breastfeeding and bathing and other rudiments of baby care. From the 1970s on, there was a worldwide trend for mothers to spend less and less time in hospital, sometimes driven by the desire of mothers to get out of an institutional setting and back to the comforts of home. This also coincided with the closure of small maternity hospitals.

But at some point that perfectly reasonable motivation overlapped with a drive to cut costs and free up hospital beds, and mothers were actively encouraged to leave as soon as possible, sometimes as little as six hours after the birth. At one point in the 1990s hospitals were offering mothers vouchers for $120 to go home earlier: the claim was that all the support and training that a new mum needs would be provided via daily visits from midwives.

Certainly the home visit approach works for some. But for many first-time mothers it didn't provide the intensity of support, especially around breastfeeding, that they get in a postnatal ward where there's a midwife there to help 24 hours a day. Even for experienced mothers, a longer hospital stay could be great – though for them it was less about learning new skills, and more about getting an enforced rest away from home before returning to the exhausting job of looking after a newborn plus another toddler or two.

As early maternal discharge became standard practice, I could see that many breastfeeding mothers were struggling. They developed mastitis (painful, inflamed breast tissue) or had poor milk supply, and would turn up at Plunket clinics or even be readmitted to hospital because their baby was losing weight. Some mothers were abandoning breastfeeding altogether, and the risk of severe post-partum depression increased.

Doctors, nurses, midwives and Plunket staff could see all this. But when it came time to do the maths, the health strategists congratulated themselves on all the beds they'd freed up. There was no line on their spreadsheet to account for the miserable women sitting at home with mastitis and a baby who wasn't feeding.

For 30-odd years I was the visiting paediatrician for a Plunket Family Centre near my home in Mt Eden. It was a low-key 'over the kitchen table' assessment of a number of babies (and mothers) who'd been identified by Plunket nurses as being in need of some help. Occasionally I'd pick up something serious – babies with severe anaemia, young children with autistic disorders, serious dyspraxias, unusual genetic syndromes, congenital heart disease or even hernias requiring surgery. But for the most part I offered reassurance and support to mothers who were struggling with feeding or were at a low ebb: for all the joys of parenthood, it's not unusual to end up exhausted, sad and lonely, especially when you're inexperienced or short of support.

It was while doing this work that I really started to question the wisdom of early maternal discharge. In many cases where infants were failing to thrive with inadequate milk supply, the problem could have been avoided if mothers had been able to establish lactation and show weight gains for their baby before discharge from the maternity unit.

Plunket itself took a hit in the budget-cutting 1990s. Since it had been founded almost a century earlier by the visionary Dr Frederic Truby King, the Royal New Zealand Plunket Society had become the country's largest provider of support services for the development, health and wellbeing of children under five. Most babies in the country were assigned a Plunket nurse who would visit several times in the first 6–12 months. Ostensibly the visits were all about the baby, but a nurse was well placed to recognise families who were in jeopardy in terms of child abuse or neglect or violence – as well as offering some general family support. Much of this was very informal – advice about budgeting or managing an older child's behaviour, say, gently delivered over a cup of tea.

As funding fell in the 1990s, Plunket had to start prioritising visits by perceived need. A mother might get more visits on the basis that she was in a low-decile suburb, didn't have a mother to offer support, and was financially struggling. But this kind of analysis is too crude; it misses, for instance, the mother in a high-decile area who has plenty of money and assets but is socially isolated because her partner works long hours and offers no support. Unless you're in that house having that cup of tea, it's hard to be certain about what you're dealing with.

This sort of false economy is rife in the health system. By the time the long-term impact from a short-sighted service cut is noticed, the management staff who've earned a bonus for slashing a budget have already moved on. No one notices initially when midwife staffing numbers are cut back at night-time, but that's because no one is actively measuring the extra misery suffered by mothers who have to wait longer for help, or the subtle social costs caused by an increase in incidences of postnatal depression.

As the health reforms started to bite, we clinicians sometimes tried to push back at unwise changes, but it was an exercise in frustration. I remember the 1990s as a time of many 'consultation' meetings: half-days put aside where medical and nursing staff sat around with a facilitator and were asked what we thought. We said what we thought, and sometimes it got pretty heated, but after a few trots around this particular block I began to realise that the plans for change were already set, and these gabfests were designed to do little more than make us feel like we were involved.

If I could wave a magic wand, I would love to get early maternal discharge rolled back. The timing of discharge from hospital after delivery should be a personal choice, and first-time mothers in particular should be warmly encouraged to stay as long as they need to get breastfeeding successfully established. Some mothers may want to get home faster than that, and that is fine, too, if we can ensure that community services are well staffed to provide all the supportive care a mother needs. My work with Brainwave has only bolstered my conviction that we must go to great lengths to ensure the first 1000 days of a child's life go as well as they can, and a lot of that is built on what happens in those first few weeks.

***

Some big changes in healthcare have been less about saving cash, and more about changing the culture. That was the case when New Zealand childbirth services underwent a major shake-up.

Through the 1990s laws were passed that gave women much more choice over whether they wanted their baby at home or in hospital, and whether the delivery would be overseen by a midwife, a GP, an obstetrician, a hospital team, or some combination of these. For uncomplicated pregnancies and labours, many women chose to have an independent midwife as their lead maternity carer (LMC). This was seen as world-leading at the time.

The push for midwives to be able to practise independently from the traditional medical system was a reaction against the 'medicalisation' of childbirth – the transition from home births to hospital births that began around 1900 and was almost total by the 1950s. Pain relief, caesarean sections and the ability of doctors to intervene if things went wrong meant childbirth became dramatically safer for both mothers and babies, but some mothers weren't so delighted by the soulless hospital environment and unnecessarily strict rules, such as banning fathers and other family members from the delivery room, or whisking perfectly healthy babies away from mothers soon after birth.

At times, the conversation about whether childbirth was the business of doctors or not became political, with overheated rhetoric on both sides. Some midwives and mothers accused doctors of being arrogant and patriarchal and far too eager to medically monitor and intervene in what was, after all, a natural process, not a disease. Doctors, meanwhile, worried that the movement against medical interventions could mean a return to the bad old days of high infant and maternal mortality.

I'm a paediatrician rather than an obstetrician, so I have always been slightly on the sidelines of this debate. When there's a high-risk birth in the hospital, I may be there at the bedside ready to assess or treat the newborn baby instantly, but the actual delivery is the responsibility of the obstetrician (and the mother, of course). All the same, it's been impossible not to develop an opinion or two about this sometimes contentious subject.

I agree that over the years there's been a tendency to pathologise or medicalise labour and delivery. For the most part, midwives do a fantastic job: by maintaining a relationship with a mother before, during and after the birth they offer great continuity of care; and there's no doubt that they can foster a low-key, supportive environment of a kind that can be lost in the hospital system.

But the important thing to remember about childbirth is that it is fundamentally unpredictable.

I remember, as a registrar at Queen Charlotte Maternity Hospital in London in the 1970s, talking to a mother who had had an emergency caesarean and whose baby had a lot of problems and was still in the neonatal unit. Everything was OK in the end, but the birth had been traumatic and the mother was still pretty shaky. As we chatted, she told me how she'd done everything right during the pregnancy: she'd eaten a perfect diet of fruit, lean meat, pulses and vegetables; she had not had a drop of alcohol or a puff of nicotine the entire nine months; and she had attended every antenatal clinic.

In the bed next to her was a younger woman who was drinking Coca-Cola and eating chips, who had smoked throughout the pregnancy, who had booked into the hospital at the last possible moment and had had virtually no antenatal care. Her baby, of course, was perfectly healthy and the birth had been trouble-free. That's just sod's law, I'm afraid. Because birth is unpredictable it pays to be ready for things to go wrong – and this is where doctors get anxious about the approach of an occasional independent midwife. There is a perception among some doctors that midwives don't recognise medical complications in pregnancy and labour when they occur because they aren't looking for them. Doctors receive training in health *and* pathology while my impression is that midwife teaching emphasises health only.

Unless a new midwife has had a year of training in a high-risk obstetric unit after graduation, it's unlikely they will have seen many (if any) instances of a birth going badly wrong – a postpartum haemorrhage where there's dangerously excessive bleeding after the birth; or an obstructed labour where a large baby's shoulders get stuck on the way out.

I have at times observed that a desire to keep things 'natural' means a midwife – or a doctor, for that matter – seems to lose sight of the main goals: the safety of mother and baby. I've got nothing against a natural delivery with soft lights, music and herbal tea, but the quality of the birth experience needs to remain a secondary consideration. Given the choice, most mothers want a healthy baby.

I talked to one mother who'd wanted a home birth but ended up delivering in hospital after things went wrong. Her baby was brain-damaged, possibly as a result. I wanted to understand what had gone wrong: obviously the decision to come into hospital had been made later than it should have.

Quite early in the labour there had been signs of meconium in the amniotic fluid, meaning that the baby has done its first poo in utero rather than waiting until she was born. This, in itself, is a warning sign of likely foetal distress, and it also creates the serious risk of meconium inhalation when the baby takes its first breath, so it should have triggered a swift move to hospital.

I asked the midwife about this and she said, 'I told the mother there's meconium present, and the mother said "I don't want to be in the hospital," so there was a bit of a delay.'

When I spoke to the mother she said, 'When the midwife saw the meconium I said, "Does this mean I have to go to hospital?" and the midwife said “Not necessarily.”” The exact truth is hard to divine, but either way, the best of intentions led to a bad decision.

Of course it’s not only midwives whose decisions look unwise in retrospect. More than once I’ve seen an obstetrician at a planned hospital birth bend over backwards to give a mother what she’s hoping for – an unimpeded natural delivery without too much monitoring and without too much intervention – and, as a result, delay longer than they should before finally announcing that it’s time to stop, divert and do an urgent caesarean.

Even when things go seriously wrong, assigning blame can be very difficult, if not impossible. A bad outcome is born of a complex mix of bad luck, bad judgement and honest error. When a childbirth goes wrong, it’s often because of the cumulative time lost during each step towards the emergency caesarean: recognising the problem in the community, admitting the mother for labour, arranging monitoring in the delivery suite, finding someone to look at the monitoring, finding an available theatre for the caesarean, performing the operation itself. At each stage, there is potential for error: someone forgets to mention that they couldn’t hear the foetal heartbeat; vital information about the mother’s health isn’t passed on. It’s not always obvious which factor mattered most, so we have a robust review process that kicks in whenever things go wrong.

I recall a case where the pregnancy seemed to be progressing fine but the obstetrics team had failed to recognise that the baby was not growing well. By the time they did, there was delay in getting the labour going. The small, already tired baby didn't cope with an induced labour and became distressed. There was an emergency caesarean and the baby began having seizures as a result of brain damage.

An investigation into this found a number of minor factors, including delay in organising the emergency delivery and finding an anaesthetist. But it also showed, from the timing of the seizures, that the brain injury most likely occurred hours before the labour and therefore the labour itself may not have been the main cause.

As midwives gained more autonomy from the 1990s on, the media reported on cases of irresponsible or even dangerous practices that had ended in tragedy. This was a time when there was an increased focus on transparency and accountability throughout the medical world, and I suspect some midwives were startled by the attention and criticism. They were learning what doctors already knew: that when things go wrong, whoever was deemed to be 'in charge' is likely to be hounded by media, regardless of whether or not there had been human error involved.

Independent midwives, in general, have excellent perinatal mortality and morbidity statistics – and so they should, given that the population they serve is selectively low-risk: if there is diabetes or high blood pressure or kidney disease or some other notable risk factor, a mother will be referred on to an obstetrician so these medical issues can be monitored.

Obstetricians are the doctors most likely to be at the sharp end of any culture clashes with midwives; and paediatricians like myself have at times been seen as the villain, too. We're the ones who take babies away from their mothers, prick them with needles and insist on regular feeding rather than the more laidback and natural 'demand feeding' if we're concerned about low weight. We're the ones who might push for a baby to be offered newborn infant formula even though we know usually 'breast is best', because we have concerns about blood sugars or hydration.

Nonetheless, the relationship between medical and midwifery staff has improved a lot since the initial shock of the 1990s reforms. Doctors are more willing to recognise the skills and abilities of both hospital and independent midwives, and midwives recognise that obstetricians are there to help out if things go wrong before and during childbirth, and that paediatricians are there if the baby then needs further help. The independent midwives are being asked to do more and more with the new mothers – talking about diet and avoidance of drugs and alcohol; showing shaken-baby videos; doing newborn blood spot tests for metabolic screening; advocating for breastfeeding; and domestic violence screening. Their job is full-on.

All the same, I still sometimes wish prospective parents were told a little bit more about the things that *can* go wrong during a pregnancy and birth. There are a number of reasons why a baby might need to be delivered by caesarean, or might arrive very early, or need a little resuscitation right after birth, or even need a stint in NICU. It would be helpful if everyone involved had a rough idea of the causes and consequences of those interventions before they needed them – and, trust me, they can't all be explained away by pointing to a paternalistic medical establishment that's itching to reach for a scalpel. We are here not because we want to take over the natural miracle of birth, but because we want to help make sure everyone gets through it alive.

CHAPTER 11

SEE ONE, DO ONE, TEACH ONE

As a teacher you have to give something of yourself: if students feel you are genuine and you care, and that teaching them isn't a chore, they are more likely to stay engaged.

The baby is deteriorating, and fast. She was born preterm a fortnight ago and has been doing well, but now she suddenly has a rising heart rate and falling oxygen saturation. The nurse spots the problem on the monitor next to the incubator and calls for a registrar, Ross, and as she waits for him she starts some more standard checks: temperature, breathing rate, the baby's colour.

When Ross arrives he's totally baffled and sensibly calls for more help. Sharon, a nurse specialist, dashes to the scene and inserts an intravenous line while junior nurse Jess hangs up the bags of fluid and starts assembling other equipment. This is looking serious, and a call is made to the consultant – who this morning happens to be me.

About three minutes later I'm at the baby's bedside. The staff here are already working well, so I step back and try to get a bird's-eye view of this unfolding crisis and think about what might be happening. Meanwhile I assign tasks: I ask Ross to take over the airway, give more oxygen and prepare to ventilate; Sharon can look after the drugs and fluids; Jess needs to record everything we're doing. The mood is busy, but still pretty calm under the circumstances.

It looks to me like the baby has a serious infection, so I request some cultures and ask Robyn, a senior nurse, to start the antibiotics. I ask for an X-ray technician but am told she is tied up, so we're going to have to make an educated guess about the condition of the baby's lungs. Just as I think we're getting on top of the situation a harried-looking nurse comes to the door: there's a bit of a situation in the next ward, and she needs Ross and Jess urgently. It's irksome, but there's nothing to be done, so we soldier on, two staff down.

With ventilation in place the oxygen saturation is lifting, and it's a relief to know the antibiotics have been successfully administered. All the same, we're still feeling anxious about the baby's fate. Which is rather curious, considering the baby is in fact a rubber mannequin and this medical 'crisis' has all been a simulation.

Though perhaps it's not all that strange that we're so caught up. Most of the equipment we're using is exactly like the real thing, right down to the monitors that are being fed fake data about the baby's status by the team running the simulation. And while the baby isn't real she is a 'high-fidelity' mannequin, so she can cry and change colour and her chest rises and falls. Her fontanelle is soft and bulges if there's excessive cranial pressure. When we try to help her breathe, her lungs won't inflate if the breathing mask seal isn't perfect or if the tube into the windpipe has been put in the wrong place.

When the scenario is called to a halt, the lesson is still only half-done. We troop into a nearby office where the five-strong simulation team is waiting to lead the debriefing. One person has been feeding the mannequin's numbers to the monitors, another has been directing the scenario including our entrances and exits, and the other three have been lurking at the edge of the room as 'qualified observers', taking note of our actions and interactions.

Sometimes, high-fidelity medical simulations like these are about practising a particular skill such as a rare surgical technique, but in this exercise we already know our individual tasks – the exercise has been about teamwork and keeping focus on the big picture even as the stresses mount. The nurse specialist and I have done this kind of thing before, but the registrar, the senior nursing sister and the three staff nurses are all newbies.

Before the exercise we introduced ourselves and did some icebreaker games – passing balls around the room faster and faster until chaos ensues, that sort of thing. Then we watched a brief video documentary about an aeroplane crash caused by communication errors in the cockpit: this, it seems, is how a series of small errors can lead to catastrophe.

Happily, our simulation didn't end in catastrophe, but the debriefing digs right down into what we did right and wrong, and especially how the team dynamic worked or didn't:

'God, I forgot to check the femoral pulses.'

'How did that happen?'

'I was thinking about something else.'

'I noticed that you hadn't checked but didn't speak up.'

'Did no one notice that the blood pressure had disappeared?'

And so on...

Ross says he felt very well supported by the senior nurses, and the junior nurses say they were pleasantly surprised to realise that their training and knowledge were up to scratch. Everyone agrees about how weird it was to become totally engaged in saving the life of a rubber doll.

Even the debrief is practice for the real world: whenever we deal with a real emergency situation, we sit down once the smoke has cleared to discuss what went right, what went wrong, and what could be done better next time.

That's exactly what we did a few months earlier after an incident involving a newborn resuscitation. This was a pregnancy that was known to be high risk because of a condition called vasa praevia, where certain major blood vessels develop in the membranes of the amniotic sac instead of inside the placenta, making them extremely vulnerable to rupture. At 31 weeks the mother suffered a huge haemorrhage; the baby was delivered in a great rush and was 'flat' – in other words requiring major resuscitation. By the time the baby had reached the NICU the situation was already looking much better – and all ended well. All the staff involved then sat down to compare notes, clarify what had happened, and ask whether there was anything to learn.

Immersive, realistic simulations of operations and other clinical events have taken off internationally in the past decade, driven by the remarkable work of a team at Boston Children's Hospital, led by Dr Peter Weinstock. Inspired by the disaster simulations that are common practice in the airline industry, they have created protocols, technologies and mannequins that allow medics to practise over and over events that would normally be so rare that a doctor or a medical team would never have the opportunity to become fluent in them. Over the past decade Auckland Hospital, like many others around the world, has benefited from the team's high-tech dolls, and their continuing research into how to improve medical practice.

At our NICU we set aside an entire morning for an exercise like this every month or two, and simulations are run in Starship's Paediatric Intensive Care Unit and elsewhere in the hospital, too. Sometimes I'm one of the simulation observers, sometimes I'm inside the simulation – and I'll confess I'm more relaxed when I'm not in the hot-seat. Research has shown that units that do this sort of inhouse training handle real-life crises better, and get better patient outcomes. It can seem like play-acting, but this stuff really works.

***

Constant learning is central to a medical career. Part of what has sustained me through nearly half a century of practice is that there is always a new theory, a new diagnostic technique, a new treatment to discover. The flipside of this is that many of us in the field remain lifelong teachers.

Formal teaching has always been one of my work responsibilities since the early 1980s – from lecturing in child and adolescent psychiatry in Oxford, to the tutoring and lecturing in paediatrics that I do for Auckland University medical students. I typically give an hour-long lecture to groups of 30 or so students every two or three weeks, and also lead smaller 'bedside' tutorials, where half a dozen students at a time come in to the ward to see what a real baby looks like. I love this teaching work, and I received a Dennis Pickup clinical educator teaching award from Auckland Hospital in 2014, and an Auckland University teaching award in 2016.

One of the challenges when lecturing to a diverse group of students is reading the room and adjusting to their learning style. Usually there are the rugby jocks who like to sit at the back of the room and wisecrack, and who sometimes need to be lured in to answering questions to prove they're actually listening. Meanwhile up at the front of the room sit the quieter students, usually female, who write down every syllable but can be reluctant to make a squeak. Over the decades the demographics have shifted: where men used to be in the majority, now it's women. Where Pākehā students once predominated, the majority of medical students now are Asian, with smaller numbers of Māori, Pasifika and other ethnicities.

I remember how excited I was in my fifth year as a medical student to finally move on from purely academic study and start to spend some time with patients. *This,* I felt, was why I had wanted to be a doctor in the first place – to have a role in the community rather than being a bottomless repository of dry information about physics and biochemistry and anatomy. Without that academic rigour, though, being a doctor would be impossible. It was at this point that I fully realised how much I appreciated the teachers who had managed to keep me engaged through those years of early study. Some teachers, in particular, managed to make the work relevant and exciting, and when I'm teaching I try to live up to the standard those teachers set.

Medicine is about relationships – and so is teaching. We know from infant neurobiology that we learn best in the context of having a relationship with our caregiver and this applies to learning, too. As a teacher you have to give something of yourself: if students feel you are genuine and you care, and that teaching them isn't a chore, they are more likely to stay engaged.

***

As much as facts, figures and technique, learning medicine is about developing the 'soft' human skills of communication, empathy, respect, body language – in short, bedside manner. This is hard to teach in the abstract, so bedside tutorials have long been at the heart of paediatric training. What you are trying to impart includes not only medical knowledge but also qualities of kindness and compassion – qualities not necessarily obtained by reading a journal or textbook.

Naturally, I need to obtain a mother's permission before bowling up with half a dozen students in tow, but if we're visiting the regular postnatal ward where the babies are mostly perfectly healthy, mothers often jump at the chance to have a senior paediatrician answer their questions.

In theory, the students already know how to do a newborn health check but, incredibly, there's always one student who's never held a baby before in their life. I demonstrate to the students how to interact with this remarkable little creature: how to swaddle; how to lift the baby up and talk to them in nonsense language; how to hold them a foot away from you at eye level and watch closely to see if they're listening; whether they're locking their gaze onto your face, and whether they're following your face as you move one way then another.

Some students are naturals. Others are embarrassed or awkward (and it would be a mistake to assume that it's always the female students who are better with babies). But they all love the interaction. Occasionally it's not a great day for the mum: perhaps milk is still coming in, or hormones and exhaustion have conspired to make her feel inexplicably tearful and sad – 'third-day baby blues'. But even then she can find it helpful to see the students' reactions and realise that other people, too, are overwhelmed by the sight of a new baby.

The babies themselves usually rise to the challenge and run the show, captivating their audience. Occasionally they'll make the day especially memorable by peeing on me or one of the students. These sessions are necessarily brief: even if we've timed it perfectly and the baby is neither hungry nor tired, they will start to weary after 10 minutes, and there's little to be gained from passing a crying infant around the room.

One part of the newborn examination – a test for hip dislocation – is saved for mannequins, as it's not great for a baby to have their limbs manipulated ineptly or repeatedly. The hip mannequins consist of the lower half of a baby – which is rather macabre, especially given the realism of the half-baby's limbs and cute little toes.

We also make bedside visits to NICU, where the physical contact with the baby is even briefer or nonexistent, and the mood can be much darker if the baby is not doing well.

One recent tutorial involved a visit to a small, sick infant – 800 grams at birth – who was on maximum ventilation but still not getting enough oxygen into her blood. For days she had been getting weaker and more miserable, and head scans showed there was already a lot of brain injury, but the parents were reluctant to consider redirection of care. This was a much-wanted child and many dreams were invested in her. They couldn't contemplate letting her go. It was remarkably generous that they gave me permission to talk about their baby with the students.

We were at the incubator only briefly, then I discussed the case with the students well away from the bedside and the parents. By the time I'd laid out the options, several of the tutorial group were speechless and pale. This was the reality of what NICU doctors and nurses have to deal with, but I had to remind myself that some of the students were only a few years out of school. They had probably seldom had a serious conversation about death and dying, let alone got involved in making decisions that might result in a baby's death.

***

There's a principle in medical training, especially for surgeons, called 'see one, do one, teach one'. It has been around since the 1890s when Johns Hopkins Hospital in Baltimore, Maryland created a residency programme that transformed the way hospitals around the world trained surgeons. The idea is simple: as a surgeon you watch once as an experienced person uses a technique; then you have a crack at it yourself under supervision; and then, seeing as you are now 'experienced' yourself, you teach it to someone else. It's a brilliant model for swiftly spreading knowledge and expertise through a system, but it has obvious flaws – including the fact that few patients want to go under the knife of someone who's never done a particular operation before.

A desire to improve on the 'see on, do one, teach one' paradigm is part of the motivation behind the increasingly sophisticated simulations that are being developed by Weinstock's team at Boston Children's Hospital. Their latest innovation goes far beyond the relatively simple mannequin-plus-software system we used in the team exercise I described earlier. With the help of computer scientists and Hollywood special-effects modelmakers, they are developing technologies that allow them to take 3D imagery of an actual brain that needs a delicate keyhole surgery – for hydrocephalus, say – and use a 3D printer to swiftly create an extraordinarily realistic model complete with rubbery brain tissue. In the hours preceding a scheduled operation, the surgical team can repeatedly practise every incision and suture on the fake brain until they feel confident enough to take a scalpel to the real patient. This is not so much 'see one, teach one, do one' as 'practise ad nauseam, *then* do one'.

When I was thrown in the deep end with my university holiday stint as house surgeon at Balclutha Hospital in the 1970s, I felt I was working to an even worse motto, something along the lines of: 'see it in a textbook, cross your fingers, give it a crack'. If there hadn't been experienced nurses on the scene to help when I was struggling, I dread to think how much worse things might have turned out.

All the same, I learnt a few important things from watching my senior colleagues in action. In London I spent almost six months doing locum shifts in the accident and emergency department at Northwick Park Hospital. During one of these shifts an elderly woman with a fractured hip arrived and I arranged for her to be admitted to hospital. Later I saw a registrar in geriatrics talking to the woman, sitting quietly holding her hand and offering sympathy and support. The registrar explained in detail everything that was going to happen, and it was as if she was talking to her own grandmother. It was a profound lesson in the importance of human kindness in a medical setting, and one I never forgot.

Back then, much on-the-job training could seem haphazard. Even little things like giving an orientation tour to every new staff member were overlooked. Whenever my London locum shifts took me to a new hospital, I made it a priority to find out the really important things the second I arrived: where the toilets were, where I would be sleeping, where the cafeteria was, and how long it would take to walk (or run) to the accident and emergency department in acute situations. I would also quickly identify which nursing sister was most likely to be an ally in telling me what to do next.

Fortunately these days, in New Zealand hospitals, the junior staff are well orientated, well supervised and mentored – and not allowed to operate independently until certain standards have been achieved under supervision.

The life of a registrar can be extraordinarily stressful as they juggle long work hours and their continuing formal study: lectures, reading related to the current cases they're managing, keeping up to date with the journals, and regular assessments. There's barely enough time in the day to meet all these demands, and an additional external pressure – a sick relative, or a young family of their own – can sometimes tip them over the edge.

At Auckland I chair the hospital Vocational Training Committee, which coordinates the work duties of our paediatric registrars with the training requirements of the College of

Paediatrics. The committee also provides support if a trainee is struggling – which more often arises from a personal crisis or stress-related burnout than from a lack of knowledge or ability.

If, say, we learn that a resident doctor has been floundering in acute situations, this could compromise clinical safety, so we'll offer a performance plan with more supervision and assessment, and an assigned mentor will also dig a bit deeper to see if there are other issues, such as a sick family member or relationship problems. If necessary, a block of training may have to be repeated.

Sometimes, though, we can see that a trainee is struggling because they're on the wrong career pathway. In those cases we have a moral duty to tell them what we think. No medical graduate wants to spend another five years of advanced training in paediatrics only to be told in the sixth and final year that they'll never make a paediatrician. We have had registrars who couldn't juggle the task of looking after several acutely sick babies at once, even though they were brilliant at handling a single complicated case. This means that they might make a very good sub-specialist in general paediatrics, but they're not cut out to specialise in intensive care.

In one extreme case things got very tricky when a young trainee refused to accept that advice. He had done his basic medical training abroad and arrived with adequate references from another New Zealand hospital, but we soon realised he was barely suited to being a clinician, let alone a paediatrician. He was frequently late to work, borrowed money from colleagues and never returned it, ran up thousands of dollars in toll calls from hospital phones, and wrote himself prescriptions for painkillers. Worse still, he'd once dumped an emergency cardiac-arrest pager before leaving the hospital rather than pass it on to the next on-call person.

This behaviour was more than unprofessional, it was unsafe; but employment law being as it is, it took us a dispiriting two years of monitoring and warnings before we were finally able to dismiss him.

***

The relationship between hospital and university isn't only about doctors like me giving lectures and tutorials for medical students. It also creates wonderful opportunities for collaborations. One research project I did alongside Auckland University professor of psychology Keith Petrie gave me a better understanding of something that was going on within my own unit.

I've always been aware that when parents first see their baby in the NICU, they can feel overwhelmed by the sheer volume of equipment encircling their child. There are wires and tubes, masks and monitors, and machines with as many dials and knobs as a 747 cockpit. Sometimes the entire scene is bathed in an uncanny blue light, because the baby has jaundice and is receiving phototherapy, where ultraviolet light striking the skin converts the yellow bilirubin molecules into safer, more easily excretable substances. Many parents find the entire setup of the ward alarming – if their baby needs all this stuff, they must be really sick! I remember one couple referring to their child's incubator as a 'glass coffin'.

Meanwhile at my private paediatric practice, when I asked for a child's early medical history I would hear from parents that years earlier their child had spent some time in NICU, where they had been at death's door. If I checked these accounts against our hospital records, I would find the parents' version of events to be distorted – their little boy had in fact needed a whiff of oxygen for a few hours and was monitored for 48 hours before being discharged in perfect health. Time and again, there would be a disconnection between parental perception and medical reality.

Keith Petrie, his masters student Stacey Brooks and I devised a piece of research to test and measure this effect. We enlisted more than 100 mothers with a baby either in NICU or the neonatal high-dependency unit (for babies that require slightly less than NICU-level care), then gave them a standardised 'illness perception' questionnaire and assessed their level of anxiety about their child. We also gave the illness perception questionnaire to the neonatologist responsible for each baby, as a kind of reality check for the parental assessments.

The results showed that whether the baby was in the unit briefly for observation or genuinely at risk of death, the parents' perception of the baby's condition, and the stress they experienced as a result, was almost exactly the same.

After the paper was published in the American journal *Health Psychology,* we tried to find ways to use the findings to improve the experience of parents who were using our services, by giving them better information about their baby's condition. In particular, we spent time with the parents of babies who were less seriously ill, giving them more-explicit reassurance that their child was going to be fine.

Funnily enough, this didn't make a lot of difference: it seems to be a parent's prerogative to regard the most important person in their life as extremely sick if they need to be taken away from them by doctors. The most useful lesson I have taken from this is that we should always be looking for ways of ensuring that mother and baby can safely be together, even if the baby has extra needs.

***

Teaching medical students and mentoring registrars on the wards keeps me on my toes: I need to keep up with the trends and technologies. Reading journal articles about the latest research is invaluable, but there's another, slightly more glamorous way to keep in touch with the wider world of paediatrics: jumping on a plane and going to a conference.

Medical conferences can be the butt of jokes; they are seen as expensive jaunts that drain the public purse to give doctors a free trip abroad. Or, perhaps worse, they're seen as junkets sponsored by 'Big Pharma' in a cynical attempt to buy doctors' allegiance to their products. As one medical blogger despairingly described a conference they'd attended, when the keynote addresses are underway 'half the audience is outside in the hallways chatting or collecting freebies', and those inside 'are fast asleep once the lights are dimmed'.

Those criticisms may contain a grain of truth at times, but personally I have drawn enormous value from the conferences I've attended over the years. At a three-day conference it's not uncommon to be in lectures, seminars or workshops from eight in the morning until 7pm. Some evenings I've emerged blinking and unsure whether I've learnt anything, but there are always a handful of things that change the way I think about our practice back in New Zealand, and which I then bring back to share with colleagues.

I was in London for the annual week-long *Neonatal Update* conference run by Imperial College London, which I try to get to every two or three years – in part to maintain my contacts with the international community of neonatologists. Events ranged from a lecture on the growing role of artificial intelligence in medicine to a masterclass in cerebral function monitoring. One standout for me was a lecture on a subject that, with any luck, will never be something we have to worry about at Auckland Hospital: war surgery. The speaker, David Nott, spends a few months every year working for Médecins Sans Frontières (Doctors Without Borders) and the British Red Cross in crisis zones such as Iraq, Afghanistan and the Darfur region of the Sudan. It was confronting stuff, including a slideshow of images of the hideous injuries that result when a bomb goes off in Aleppo or Basra, in Kabul or Sierra Leone. Nott made the point that the biggest casualties of war, both physically and psychologically, are children. I was especially stunned by the video he played of an emergency caesarean delivery for a woman who had been shot in the abdomen by a sniper. The bullet went through the uterus but missed the baby – who filled his lungs and gave a healthy yell the moment he was delivered.

In previous years at this same conference I've heard a lecture by Robert Winston about the ethics of assisted fertility, learnt about the latest obesity research, and heard from researchers who are sequencing the newborn genome in the hope of detecting serious conditions long before they become apparent.

In the last 5–10 years neonatology researchers have made huge strides in understanding how our environment during gestation, and even before conception, has the power to determine the course of our entire life, and at most conferences I hear some new variation on this theme. It seems that even at the age of 70 our physical health may have been partly determined by what our mother ate while pregnant and what we were exposed to in the womb. This has some scary implications, but it creates opportunities to see what we can do to get things right – for future generations at least.

I always encourage trainee paediatricians to travel before they settle down back here at home – roam the world with a backpack or, if they're too career-focused for that, I suggest they take a diploma in infectious diseases at the Liverpool School of Tropical Medicine or do some volunteer aid work in a developing country, or work for a while in another country's healthcare system. My experiences in Oxford and at Great Ormond Street Hospital in London helped me realise that the standard of paediatrics in New Zealand is pretty damn good. I was impressed, however, by how my bosses who had written the definitive text in physiology or paediatric diagnosis would still be asking questions, and be prepared to phone colleagues for a second opinion about a puzzling child. In New Zealand we had tended to rely on our own knowledge. Canvassing our colleagues for opinions is now part of everyday practice.

***

I give 30 or so lectures a year to med students, but one of the great things about a teaching hospital is that teaching is woven into the everyday rhythms of work. The registrar system – where junior paediatricians cycle through our ward in stints of four to six months – means that the unit is also a classroom. The ward's nurse specialists (who operate at a similar clinical level to registrars) and regular nurses are teaching and learning on the job as well.

As a senior clinician I'm always quietly modelling soft skills such as the way we interact with staff and parents. If I'm about to break some tough news to parents, I'll usually take a registrar and nurse with me so they're familiar with the mood of these situations long before they have to be the bearer of bad news themselves.

And remember that ward round from the opening pages of this book, where the registrar Logan outlines his intentions for the babies' treatment and I offer questions and suggestions as we move from incubator to incubator? That's not simply a staff member reporting to a boss. It's also a lesson – part of the endless dialectic that plays out every day in thousands of hospitals around the world between a grizzled consultant (literally, in my case; there's a lot of grey in my beard) and the trainee doctors and nurses who are still soaking up knowledge like a sponge.

It's a kind of investigation, too, as we all – the consultant, the registrars, the specialist nurse, the nurses – talk our way through the mysteries of our work.

The second-to-last baby we see that day has us stumped. She was born at 25 weeks' gestation and was doing well until she got a nasty cytomegalovirus infection – a virus that causes a flulike illness in adults, and can be devastating for a baby if it's transferred to the foetus in utero, or if a preterm baby catches it. She then developed pneumonia, requiring a return to ventilation. She's almost stable again now, but has puzzlingly high sodium levels in her blood (hypernatraemia). She seems to be coping OK, but in extreme cases hypernatraemia can cause seizures, so we will need to sort this soon.

She's quietly mewling and unsettled, even though her mother is by the incubator, gently patting her nappied bottom. We gather in a huddle at the other side of the incubator, collectively musing over the sodium. Is she getting too much salt in her food? Are we giving her enough water? Does she have a kidney or adrenal problem? Has one of the drugs we gave her to combat the virus caused this? What do the endocrinologists say about her thyroid function? Diuretics would help her lose some sodium in her urine, but that could dehydrate her, so we'd need to get more water on board too. It's not yet urgent, but definitely needs resolving.

The baby is still a bit restless, so I move back to the incubator. I hope the mother is noticing what I'm about to do, because her gentle but anxious patting of the baby is the exact opposite of what's needed.

The little girl is tiny, her whole body roughly the size of my hand. I place her on her back and, without lifting her, firmly envelop her entire body in my cupped hands and murmur something comforting. The feeling of physical security and support – maybe an echo of the pressure inside the womb – calms her instantly and she stops crying. Using two thumbs so I don't need to release my cupped hands, I wiggle a tiny dummy back into her mouth. She starts sucking, and after 30 seconds or so I gingerly release her from my swaddling hands. As we walk towards the final incubator, chatting about the rogue sodium numbers, I glance back and can see she's still sucking, and has closed her eyes.

CHAPTER 12

A GOOD HARD STARE

As a paediatrician I've been able to enjoy, over and over again, pleasures that most people only experience a handful of times with their own children or those of friends and family.

My home is in the shadow of Maungawhau/Mt Eden, and for a long time I used to get up early every morning, cross the street and and climb to the summit, often with my son's dog Dexter. I like to be up there before anyone else, so I can hear the quiet of the sleeping city before the traffic hum and groups of chatty joggers start.

Every October the shining cuckoos – the pīpīwharauroa – arrive from Indonesia and start evicting the eggs from the nests of the grey warblers (riroriro) to make room for their own parasitic offspring. Some years I reckon I've been the first person in the city to hear these beautiful little freeloaders announcing their return from their winter break: three rising notes then a series of chittering downward swoops.

Of late, I've been getting up the hill only every couple of weeks. My hip surgeon said I should avoid too much downhill walking, and though I toyed with the idea of carrying a trolley or skateboard to the top then freewheeling home, I never quite did.

But this morning, a Saturday in early December, I'm feeling fit and I'm up very early anyway, still a little jetlagged from the London neonatal conference. I'm technically at work – I've been the on-call consultant since the previous evening – but it's been a quiet night and the cellphone in my pocket will let me know if I need to rush in before the scheduled ward round at 8.30am.

Rather than head direct to the summit, I take a detour through a small park at the base of the volcano. About 15 years ago I snuck in and did some guerilla gardening to fill in some gaps in the stand of bush along the park perimeter, and I like to see how my babies are coming along. The council's drive to repopulate Auckland parks with native species is laudable, but seems rather fixated on pōhutukawa and a few varieties of pittosporum and coprosma, so I quietly increased the biodiversity by smuggling in a dozen or so different saplings: pūriri, karaka, kahikatea, toru, wharangi, tawa, tītoki, tawāpou and more. Some of them are now getting on for five metres in height. They're looking splendid.

I take the road that gently spirals clockwise towards the summit, and as I get higher the familiar shapes of Auckland are revealed: uneven stripes of green land and shining water, and volcanoes in every direction. Over to the southeast, at the foot of Maungakiekie/One Tree Hill, is the old National Women's Hospital, where I spent my first 20 years as a paediatric consultant. The hospital overlooked the fields of Cornwall Park, and I used to watch the grazing sheep, reputedly the very same ewes who'd borne the lambs used by Graham Liggins for his famous research into foetal lung development.

Just to the east is Ōhinerau/Mt Hobson, a vigorous stone's throw from my former paediatric clinic in Remuera. To the north is my current workplace, Auckland Hospital, which is built literally on *top* of a volcano – though to be fair, the 45,000-year-old scoria cone of Grafton Volcano was so well buried it wasn't identified as such until building excavations unearthed it in the 1990s. The hospital complex is identifiable from a distance by the towering incinerator chimney next to the main building.

***

When I was a registrar at John Radcliffe Hospital in Oxford in the 1980s, one of my teachers was the professor of paediatrics Peter Tizard, an intimidatingly distinguished man who was knighted a few years later (I learnt afterwards that his father, also a sir, had helped design the UK's radar system during the Second World War, invented the octane rating system for petrol, and led the UK's first serious investigation into UFOs).

Anyway, once while we were examining a baby during a ward round, one of my colleagues asked Tizard a question: 'We've done the tests to assess this child's neurological state, but how do you assess his *intellectual* state?'

Tizard paused for a moment, then said: 'I think probably the best measure of that is if a child gives you a good hard stare.'

Tizard and I didn't get on terribly well – I got the feeling he always viewed me as an antipodean upstart – but that small, commonsense observation has stayed with me. There is nothing quite like the feeling you get when a newborn child locks you in her gaze – it's a reassuring sign that there's plenty going on behind those pupils of bottomless black.

There is something intense, almost sombre, about a healthy newborn, and that's not only because she's still a month or two away from her first smile. It's not fanciful to imagine that this child is conducting an investigation of the person who's looking at her:

Who the hell are you?

Do I know you?

Are you a good person?

Investigating you is precisely what she's doing as she sets about the huge project of adapting herself to the world, as well as adapting the world to herself. As any new parent knows, the real power in this early relationship lies with the helpless creature who on the face of it can do little more than sleep, eat, poo and cry.

As a paediatrician I've been able to enjoy, over and over again, pleasures that most people only experience a handful of times with their own children or those of friends and family.

In the first few weeks of a baby's life there's plenty of fun to be had with a baby's mirroring behaviour, as they observe, then try to reflect back, the expression on the face of their carer (though sometimes it's hard to tell whether the poking tongue and furrowed brow are deliberate or a side effect of straining to fill a nappy).

By four to six weeks, you can expect the first smile. This is an important milestone and missing it can be an early warning of a developmental delay, so I've had a number of consultations where the matter at hand is 'baby hasn't smiled yet'.

Often the baby is ready to smile – they just haven't had quite the encouragement they need. I demonstrate to parents how to move things along by hamming it up: screw up your face, poke out your tongue, give a big smile of your own, make some coos and gagas and peekaboos and get up in your baby's face, and see what happens next. Once or twice I've managed to extract that first smile there and then in my office – the smallest but most rewarding clinical success you could imagine. This approach to a newborn baby was a particular skill demonstrated by a famous US paediatrican, Dr Berry Brazelton, who is one of my heroes in neonatology.

Some of these cases did, however, involve a mother who was suffering from postnatal depression and genuinely struggling to crack a smile of her own, so the long-term solution involved a bit more than an ad hoc lesson in clowning.

In the course of my work I've been witness to the first (or an early) instance of a giggle, a successful rolling over, a pushup and a handclap; of coos and gaas, bubble-blowing, crawling and first steps. Through childhood and all the way into adolescence there are firsts and milestones, and it's always a pleasure to share in them.

With premature babies the calendar is timeshifted by their early arrival, so we talk about 'adjusted age' – the age a child would be if they'd been born at full term. During those weeks or months in NICU where the adjusted age is still less than zero, the milestones we celebrate are fundamentally different from those of a full-termer: rather than a wise stare or a chortle, we'll settle for a safe level of jaundice or a stable respiration pattern without ventilation. Yet even this early there are glimmers of individual personality, and you can distinguish the stroppy movers from the quiet observers.

Very early on, the youngest premature babies don't even look entirely human. Some remind me of tiny piglets, and those who are born with a full-body coat of lanugo – a fine downy hair that grows on the foetus in utero but is usually shed at around eight months – are like cute little woodland creatures. (I'm always careful to assess the parental sense of humour before I start suggesting that someone's baby looks like a pig or a rabbit. The responses can go either way.)

All this means that when a premature baby has done their catching up in NICU and been discharged home for a month or two, it's a double thrill when the family come back in for a check-up and I discover this furry creature has been transformed into a bonny, age-adjusted six-week-old who's now beaming at me from the pram.

It probably took me longer than it should have to realise that an obsession with milestones can interfere with seeing the individual child behind the measurements.

One of the reasons parents come to a paediatrician is because they worry that their child is different from their peers, or seems slow or 'abnormal'. But the more children I've seen, the more I love meeting those who *are* different or eccentric or quirky. I'm intrigued by those who are ahead of their milestones and those who are behind; by those with tics and unusual obsessions; by those with jiggling legs and inexhaustible energy, or a physical difference that will shape their life. In some cases I feel that my biggest achievement for a child has been to talk with the parents and help them realise that when it comes to *this* child, 'different' is totally OK.

***

Just before the summit, the path skirts the rim of Maungawhau's volcanic cone – a deep, steep, grass-lined parabolic bowl. The path cuts through long grass that's gone to seed and I recognise all the pasture grasses from my farm childhood: Yorkshire fog, fescue, Timothy, ryegrass, cocksfoot, browntop. I love the rich, promising smell of grass at this time of year –

you can tell it's ready to be cut and made into hay.

It's getting noisy as the shining cuckoos and grey warblers compete for airtime as well as nest occupancy, and the tūī are joining in too. It's the middle of the breeding season; many of the tūī are still very young and their songs are plain – just a few bells and gongs rather than the beat-box polyphony of an adult. Like us humans, they take a while to complete their brain development and learn all the important life skills.

From up here you realise that Auckland is really quite green, not the tarmac tangle it sometimes seems when you're nose-to-tail on a motorway. To the northeast, the Harbour Bridge straddles the channel between Point Erin and Northcote Point. I don't make it to the North Shore very often, but one night after an especially gruelling shift that ended in the wee hours I got in my car for the short drive home and the radio was tuned to my favourite FM country station. A Tammy Wynette song came on and I really wanted to hear it to the end, so I swung onto the motorway and roared across the bridge with Tammy blaring, looped around at the Takapuna motorway exit and back over the bridge again – a highly effective tension reliever that I repeated a few times after that.

I've come to love this city the best, despite growing up in the country and living for extended periods in Dunedin, Christchurch and Wellington.

There was a brief period though, after I returned to New Zealand in 1975 following a couple of years of travel, when I felt disenchanted with the entire country.

In the northern hemisphere I'd worked in several London hospitals, hitchhiked across North Africa with a friend, taken a campervan through Scandinavia, roamed the Greek Islands, and lived in Italy for ages, including three months studying Italian at the Università per Stranieri in Perugia. I'd visited galleries, made friends and learnt new ways to do medicine. But when I fetched up back in Christchurch as a registrar, several people asked me if I'd enjoyed my 'holiday', and I felt a kind of despair about the insularity of New Zealand life. Suddenly everything about the place irritated me: the harshness of the light, the clarity of the air, the lack of people, the empty roads and hopeless public transport, the wantonly mismatched buildings, the corrugated iron – even the sound of rain on a tin roof was offensive to my newly cosmopolitan ears.

Of course those are the exact things that endear New Zealand to many of us, and in time I came down to earth and stopped feeling sorry for myself. It probably helped that it was around this time I met Ann at a dinner with mutual friends. She'd not long returned from Europe as well, and had by chance also studied in Perugia, so we loved going out to the local Italian restaurants and practising our Italian.

We have travelled plenty since, but it was around then that we realised New Zealand was going to be home in the long run, and I knew that one way or another my career would involve working with babies and children.

When I set my sights on paediatrics I had no idea that shifts in technology and technique would mean we could get quite so good at saving younger and younger babies. I didn't know that in the older children I saw, ADHD and autism diagnoses would soar, or that an old drug called methylphenidate would get a new lease of life as the miracle ADHD pill Ritalin. I didn't know that DNA technologies would transform the diagnosis of genetic disorders, or that we would learn so much about the significance of childhood trauma in brain development. What I intuited, though, was that this was a field where there would always be new things to learn, and in this I've never been disappointed.

In paediatrics, the effects of much of your work isn't fully apparent until decades later. An immunisation programme for infectious diseases isn't only keeping children healthy right now; it's protecting them from long-term effects – the liver cancer or cirrhosis that sometimes kicks in 50 years after a hepatitis B infection, or the lifelong disabilities caused by meningitis.

We know that improvements in a child's environment in their first 1000 days will resonate throughout their lifetime and that of their children. We know that good nutrition during pregnancy, breastfeeding rather than bottle-feeding, parental smoking cessation and improvements in housing quality will all confer benefits that will still be measurable in 20 or 40 or 60 years' time. Like my guerilla tree planting, it's nice to think that some of the work you and your colleagues do will still count, even after you're gone.

There's an individualised version of that, too: when you work with babies, you're liable to keep bumping into your patients for the rest of your life.

A couple of months ago I was called to the hospital reception to see a visitor. Her name was Tamryn, and when my colleague Jean and I first met her she was a 25-weeker weighing 620 grams. We remembered Tamryn despite the passage of years because her case had been medically a little unusual: she'd had septicaemia that took several days to respond to antibiotics, and she also suffered an injury to her nose because of the way we taped the endotracheal ventilation tube to her face. At time of discharge we were still quite anxious about her prospects.

At reception that day it was obvious that our fears hadn't been realised. Tamryn is now a healthy, successful 32-year-old with a university degree, and the reason she wanted to see us this day in particular was so she could introduce us to her husband – and their beautiful boy, born full-term at a healthy 3.6 kilograms.

Tamryn had visited once a few years earlier, but this time Jean, one of our senior nurses, was passing and I stopped her to reintroduce her to Tamryn.

'Oh I remember you well,' she said. 'I spent many, many hours at your bedside looking after you.' Tamryn teared up, and to be honest, so did the rest of us.

Tamryn is not the only graduate who pops in with a progress report. Last year I gave a tour of the NICU to twins, now in their late teens, who'd been born at 28 weeks' gestation: they were on their way to Dunedin where the boy was about to start med school and his sister was in her second year of primary teacher training.

One letter we received in the NICU last year captures the experience from the parents' point of view with such elegance and clarity that I asked the mother, Madeleine Tobert, if she would mind me reproducing it, and she generously agreed.

2 August 2017

Dear Doctors and NPs [Nurse Practitioners],

When your waters break at 17 weeks, people don't talk to you about your baby; they talk to you about how to handle your miscarriage. For eight long weeks of leaking and bleeding, I was told how it might happen, what to expect and even offered an abortion to make the whole thing easier. And then at

23 weeks 5 days, I was allowed into hospital and there was a chance that something might be done if, if, if ... always if. Until Anna came to see us from NICU and then the conversation changed.

Don't get me wrong, she didn't paint a rosy picture and certainly didn't promise a future for that little dot of mine, but she did talk about what we might expect once that baby came out. The baby. Not the miscarriage, the baby. And when she asked what she was called Save and I told her what we were playing with – Elenoa. It was Anna who used her name for the first time and suddenly Ellie was real; we were having a baby.

Anna asked what kind of people we were – did we want to know everything, all the details, all the possibilities or just get a big picture? I had no idea but Save confidently answered, 'Tell us everything', and she did. And it was emotional and overwhelming and while we tried to ask sensible medical questions, at that stage there was only one that really interested me: 'Are you guys awesome? Have you got this?'

'We're awesome,' she replied.

She was right. You saved my baby. You're awesome.

It's just impossible to thank you for that in a way that is at all meaningful. Cheers, much appreciated. It all sounds ridiculous! But nonetheless thank you.

Thank you for knowing what to do with a 650 gram human who couldn't breathe. Thank you for ventilating her, drugging her, putting all those lines in and dealing with her pneumothorax while I lay drugged and useless and Save prowled the corridors.

Thank you for steroids. For knowing that those were the things that might turn her around when fiddling with the ventilator settings wasn't doing much, her oxygen requirements continued to climb and it looked like she wasn't too keen to hang around.

(Thanks for all the study you must have done to gain the knowledge you used on Ellie. Committing to learning and continuing to learn actual real information, with real lifesaving application is something that never even crossed my mind! What you do is humbling.)

Thanks for being straight with us. Save was right. We are people who want to know everything. And it was good to know how bad things were when they were bad. Thanks for being honest and for drip-feeding us ideas so that nothing came as a shock. And thanks for all the lessons. Miraculously, I feel like I've understood all the twists and turns of Ellie's journey and never got lost in the medicine. As I have exactly no science, that's a great testament to your explanations.

Thank you for NIPPV [non-invasive positive pressure ventilation]. For CPAP. For high-flow. For getting her off the ventilator and onto something better, something less. We're now happily home on low-flow. Thanks for moving that process along.

Thank you for drugs. For iron, Vitadol C, zinc, caffeine, fortifier, Labinic, dex, Nitrex, morphine, even sucrose and whatever other good stuff you pumped her with. I laugh now thinking about what a purist I was with my first daughter. No caffeine, no sugar for me, no medicine for her. But Ellie's needs were different. Thanks for catering to them.

Thank you for blood transfusions, and for stern words when the first one freaked me out. Ellie had six in the end. Thanks for the phrase 'let's optimise her', which changed the visual from '90s British documentaries of '80s tainted blood, to Energizer bunny positivity.

Thanks for not being all work, all the time. You guys were also our entire social life for most of this year so small conversations about your kids, holidays, weddings, mutual friends, even earaches, made days less abnormal, made hospital life almost fun.

Thanks for getting to know Elenoa. For really taking the time to know not just her lungs, her head rash, her hernia, her checklist of medical problems, but also her little personality – her fight, her sass, her moods, her ways of telling us what's happening with her. Whenever anyone talked to her directly to say hello or check in, I melted inside. It may have been a small thing to you but it meant everything to us.

I keep thinking of more things to thank you for but this has already turned into an essay so I better stop the list there. All those other things you did that I haven't written about, I saw them, appreciate them and all of it more than I can ever convey. Honestly. Really. Thank you for Ellie.

The baby in question is now fast asleep is our bedroom, being tube fed by her daddy. It's 10pm. We've spent the day cuddling and breastfeeding and doing other normal newborn things – nappies, pictures and some slightly less common things – drugs and oxygen tanks. But the important thing is we've done them here.

My baby is home. And that's because of all of you.

Thank you.

Madeleine, Savenaca and Elenoa.

How could anyone in the NICU team read a letter like this and not feel happy about their career choice?

Of all the reconnections with past neonates, the saddest was in 2004 when Joshua Robinson who, along with his twin Tabitha, had spent three months in NICU at National Women's Hospital, drowned at the age of seven while swimming in the supposedly safe waters of Browns Bay on Auckland's North Shore. The twins' older sister Christie, plus an adult woman who had swum out to help the children when they got into trouble, also drowned. It was a shocking tragedy, and I was very touched when Joshua's parents asked me to say a few words at the funeral about the twins' time in our care.

***

By the time I reach the summit of Maungawhau the phone in my pocket still hasn't rung, but there's no guarantee it will stay quiet. Just over there, in the hospital that's built on a buried volcano, there are two women threatening very early delivery, each of them just far enough through pregnancy to put their baby on the cusp of viability.

For one of the babies a delivery today would probably be survivable, but the other baby needs to stay where it is for at least a couple of days longer to get on the right side of the fine line between miscarriage and extreme prematurity.

The mothers are in the hands of highly qualified obstetricians who have a few tricks for slowing down a process that's starting way too early – but the experts aren't really running this show. The time of delivery will be determined by a million little interrelated biochemical processes; or, to put it another way, the babies will come when they're good and ready. When that happens the obstetrics team will get them through it, and then the NICU team will be there to try to give the new arrivals a shot at life. It could all kick off any minute, or it could be days away. It may turn out OK; it may not.

Doctors often get accused of wanting to play God, but in NICU – the area of my career where the team makes truly life-and-death decisions – we know we have only limited control over how things turn out.

As I walk back down the hill (slowly, as per the hip surgeon's instructions), I can't help thinking of one of the babies we'd seen during that Thursday evening ward round I described earlier. Born extremely early, she was the last of the 14 babies we saw that day, and she was a source of constant surprises. Before birth, scans showed she had very serious cardiac and gut problems, and based on the advice we gave, the parents decided they would rather let nature take its course after birth. She arrived, and as planned, we offered palliative care – the bare minimum treatment required to keep her comfortable, with the expectation of imminent death.

This little girl, however, had other plans. Over her first three days she proved surprisingly vigorous, and kept demanding more care and attention. This was a baby who seemed to want to live. We talked to the parents, reassessed the options and arranged for a corrective bowel surgery, which went well. Now, she was recovering in an NICU incubator.

We gathered round, and Logan summarised her status and the treatment intentions for the coming day. The numbers on Logan's chart looked good, and so did she: she was napping, and beneath the mask and tubes her skin had a healthy colour and her expression was calm.

At some point soon, she would need heart surgery. We wouldn't know for a while what harm, if any, had occurred during the period of palliative care, when her glucose levels and electrolytes weren't closely managed. There were still obstacles ahead, but she had already proven herself a fighter, and that counted for a lot.

Logan's plans sounded about right to me, so there wasn't much more to say. We each took a final glance at the sleeping girl and quietly left the room.

GLOSSARY

ALVEOLUS tiny sac that allows for gas exchange in lungs

ASPERGER'S SYNDROME high-functioning autism

AUTISM SPECTRUM DISORDER range of autism from severe to mild

COT DEATH (SUDDEN INFANT DEATH SYNDROME) sudden unexpected death in infancy

CYTOMEGALOVIRUS (CMV) INFECTION flu-like illness due to CMV virus

DOWN SYNDROME (TRISOMY 21) caused by extra copy of chromosome 21

ENDOCRINOLOGIST doctor specialising in diseases of endocrine glands

EPIGENETICS study of how genes are switched on/off

HYPERNATRAEMIA high blood sodium level

HYPONATRAEMIA low blood sodium level

IMPETIGO 'school sores' caused by bacteria

METHYLPHENIDATE stimulant drug used to treat ADHD

MOEBIUS SYNDROME absence of/damage to nerves supplying face

MYELINATION fatty coating of nerve fibres

NEURON nerve cell

PERINATAL ASPHYXIA lack of oxygen and blood to brain around birth

PREFRONTAL CORTEX front part of the brain – enables rational thinking

PRUNING reduction of excess nerve fibres not in use

RETICULAR FORMATION part of brain controlling basic functions, e.g. pulse

SYNAPSES connections between neurons

TERATOGEN substance causing malformation of foetus in utero

ABBREVIATIONS

ACC	Accident Compensation Corporation
ACE	adverse childhood experience
ADHD	attention deficit and hyperactivity disorder
ASD	autism spectrum disorder
CDC	Centers for Disease Control and Prevention
CPAP	continuous positive airway pressure
CYF	Child, Youth and Family
FAS	foetal alcohol syndrome
FASD	foetal alcohol spectrum disorder
HEADDSS	health, education, activities, drugs, depression, sex, suicide
HIB	Haemophilus influenzae type B (vaccine)
LMC	lead maternity carer
MMR	measles, mumps and rubella (vaccine)
MCOT	Ministry for Children Oranga Tamariki
NICU	Newborn Intensive Care Unit
RDS	respiratory distress syndrome

ACKNOWLEDGEMENTS

To my wife, Ann, who has never once complained about the intrusion of work on my private life and who has quietly reminded me not to totally neglect my own children.

To my children, Joe, Patrick, Tom and Francesca, and their friends, all of whom keep me down to earth.

To my medical and nursing colleagues over the years, too many to name, at both Auckland City Hospital and Starship Children's Hospital – the best team ever to work with, and always there to support and encourage each other when things are busy and stressful. Such collegiality in medicine, especially in intensive care, is what prevents burnout and ensures that we remain enthusiastic and keen to come to work.

To the editorial staff at Penguin Random House, who have been enthusiastic about this project, and to my 'ghost writer', Adam Dudding, who painstakingly edited tapes and rewrote passages into a palatable form with intelligence, humour and patience.

Last but not least, to my patients – the babies and children, who are such great teachers, and their parents, who have demonstrated true selfless devotion to their children. Their resilience and strength never fail to amaze me.

The little 'survivor' described in the final pages of this book successfully negotiated major heart surgery in February 2018 and was doing well but, sadly, died suddenly a week later. I am grateful to her parents for allowing us to include her in the book.

ABOUT THE CO-AUTHOR

Adam Dudding is a senior reporter for Stuff and has won numerous national journalism awards, including Newspaper Feature Writer of the Year at the 2013 Canon Media Awards. He was previously on the staff of the *Guardian*, the *Independent* and the *Independent on Sunday* in the United Kingdom.

His literary memoir *My Father's Island* won the E.H. McCormick award for Best First Non-Fiction Book at the 2017 Ockham New Zealand Book Awards.

Adam lives in Auckland with his wife, two children and a dog.

www.ingramcontent.com/pod-product-compliance
Lightning Source LLC
LaVergne TN
LVHW031614210926
848480LV00011B/1483
* 9 7 8 1 5 2 5 2 7 5 9 2 0 *